Pathophysiologic Basis of Acid-Base Disorders

Farrokh Habibzadeh • Mahboobeh Yadollahie
Parham Habibzadeh

Pathophysiologic Basis of Acid-Base Disorders

Springer

Farrokh Habibzadeh
Petroleum Industry Health Organization
Shiraz
Iran

Mahboobeh Yadollahie
Petroleum Industry Health Organization
Shiraz
Iran

Parham Habibzadeh
Persian BayanGene Research
and Training Center
Shiraz
Iran

ISBN 978-981-16-0525-3 ISBN 978-981-16-0526-0 (eBook)
https://doi.org/10.1007/978-981-16-0526-0

This Springer imprint is published by the registered company Springer Nature Singapore Pte Ltd.
The registered company address is: 152 Beach Road, #21-01/04 Gateway East, Singapore 189721, Singapore

Preface

"In teaching the medical student, the primary requisite is to keep him/her awake."

Chevalier Jackson (1865–1958)

During our medical clerkship, we were feeling the lack of an appropriate text on acid-base disorders. Later on, we found several books on the topic. Nevertheless, we found none of them appropriate for medical students; the books were either too detailed and lengthy to be used by a medical student who has a limited amount of time, or too simple and concise to meet the needs of daily practice. This turned a wheel in our mind to develop a proper text that we were long looking for—simple, concise, and informative.

This book consists of nine chapters. It is assumed that the reader has only a very basic knowledge of mathematics, chemistry, and medical terminology. We, therefore, decided to start from the scratch. The first four chapters deal with the basic knowledge necessary for understanding the clinical concepts, which are explained in Chapters 5–9. The material explored in each section is further clarified by several examples throughout the text.

Although we have tried to prepare an error-free text, we are sure that an astute reader may pick up many errors. The authors welcome all relevant critiques and appreciate your correspondence.

We would like to thank all who have helped us in numerous ways in preparing this book. Finally, we hope this book keeps all the medical students who read it awake.

Shiraz, Iran — Farrokh Habibzadeh, MD
Shiraz, Iran — Mahboobeh Yadollahie, MD
Shiraz, Iran — Parham Habibzadeh, MD
November 2020

Contents

About the Author

Farrokh Habibzadeh is a general practitioner and author of more than 150 peer-reviewed articles and 6 book chapters. He has been involved in biomedical research, scientific writing, and editorship craft since 30 years ago. He was the Editor of *The International Journal of Occupational and Environmental Medicine* for 11 years.

Mahboobeh Yadollahie is a general practitioner and author of more than 50 peer-reviewed articles and 3 book chapters. She has been involved in biomedical research and scientific writing since 15 years ago. She was the Deputy Editor of *The International Journal of Occupational and Environmental Medicine* for 11 years.

Parham Habibzadeh graduated from Shiraz University of Medical Sciences with first class honors. He is the author of more than 40 peer-reviewed articles and has received many national and international awards including an Honorary Diploma from the Iranian Academy of Medical Sciences. Currently, he is the Director of the R&D Department, Persian BayanGene Research and Training Center.

1 Starting from Scratch

It's elementary, Watson

Sherlock Holmes

1.1 Calculation with Powers

When we say, $A = 5^3$ (read "five raised to the power of three"), we mean that 5 is to be multiplied 3 times by itself. Thus:

$$A = 5 \times 5 \times 5$$

In general, if we have $A = B^p$, B is called the "base," and p is named the "power," "exponent," or "index."

Example

$$6.02^3 = 6.02 \times 6.02 \times 6.02$$
$$7^4 = 7 \times 7 \times 7 \times 7$$

1.1.1 Multiplication and Division of Numbers Having the Same Base, *B*

If $N = B^6$ and $M = B^2$, then:

$$\begin{aligned} N \times M &= B^6 \times B^2 \\ &= (B \times B \times B \times B \times B \times B) \times (B \times B) \\ &= B \times B \times B \times B \times B \times B \times B \times B \\ &= B^8 \\ &= B^{6+2} \end{aligned}$$

F. Habibzadeh et al., *Pathophysiologic Basis of Acid-Base Disorders*,
https://doi.org/10.1007/978-981-16-0526-0_1

In general, if the numbers have the same base (here, B), *powers must be added*. Thus:

$$B^p \times B^q = B^{p+q}$$

Example

$$2^3 \times 2^4 = 2^{3+4} = 2^7$$
$$3^1 \times 3^9 = 3^{1+9} = 3^{10}$$
$$0.5^7 \times 0.5^2 = 0.5^{7+2} = 0.5^9$$

In a similar way, if $N = B^6$ and $M = B^2$, then:

$$\begin{aligned}\frac{N}{M} = \frac{B^6}{B^2} &= \frac{B \times B \times B \times B \times B \times B}{B \times B} \\ &= B \times B \times B \times B \\ &= B^4 \\ &= B^{6-2}\end{aligned}$$

In general, if the numbers have the same base, the power of the denominator must be subtracted from that of the numerator, and we can write:

$$\frac{B^p}{B^q} = B^{p-q}$$

Example

$$\frac{B^4}{B^3} = B^1 = B$$
$$\frac{0.75^6}{0.75^2} = 0.75^{6-2} = 0.75^4$$
$$\frac{10.1^3}{10.1} = \frac{10.1^3}{10.1^1} = 10.1^{3-1} = 10.1^2$$

Example Now let us find the results of the following divisions:

$$A = \frac{3^4}{3^4}$$

Solution: The numerator and denominator are equal and thus:

$$A = \frac{3 \times 3 \times 3 \times 3}{3 \times 3 \times 3 \times 3} = 1$$

but, according to our general rule, we have:

$$A = \frac{3^4}{3^4} = 3^{4-4} = 3^0$$

Therefore, $3^0 = 1$.

$$C = \frac{B^p}{B^p}$$

Solution:

$$C = \frac{B^p}{B^p} = 1$$

because the numerator equals the denominator, but employing the general rule for division, we have:

$$C = \frac{B^p}{B^p} = B^{p-p} = B^0$$

Therefore, it can be stated that *any non-zero number raised to the power of zero equals one*, that is:

$$B^0 = 1$$

$$D = \frac{3^3}{3^5}$$

Solution:

$$\begin{aligned} D = \frac{3^3}{3^5} &= \frac{3\times3\times3}{3\times3\times3\times3\times3} \\ &= \frac{1}{3\times3} \\ &= \frac{1}{3^2} \end{aligned}$$

but, using our general rule, we have:

$$D = \frac{3^3}{3^5} = 3^{3-5} = 3^{-2}$$

Therefore:

$$3^{-2} = \frac{1}{3^2}$$

$$F = \frac{1}{B^p}$$

Solution: Using what we have learned earlier, and substituting B^0 for 1, the above division can be rewritten as:

$$\begin{aligned} F = \frac{1}{B^p} &= \frac{B^0}{B^p} \\ &= B^{0-p} \\ &= B^{-p} \end{aligned}$$

Therefore:

$$\frac{1}{B^p} = B^{-p}$$

Example

$$\begin{aligned}\frac{1}{3^4} &= 3^{-4} \\ \frac{1}{0.6^3} &= 0.6^{-3} \\ \frac{1}{0.8^3 \times 0.8^{-3}} &= \frac{1}{0.8^{[3+(-3)]}} \\ &= \frac{1}{0.8^0} \\ &= \frac{1}{1} = 1\end{aligned}$$

1.1.2 Powers Raised to Powers

Example

$$\begin{aligned}\left(5^2\right)^3 &= 5^2 \times 5^2 \times 5^2 \\ &= (5\times5)\times(5\times5)\times(5\times5) \\ &= 5\times5\times5\times5\times5\times5 \\ &= 5^6 \\ &= 5^{2\times3}\end{aligned}$$

In general, we have:

$$\left(B^p\right)^q = B^{p\times q}$$

Example If we have:

$$A = 125^{\frac{1}{3}}$$

raising both sides to the power of 3 gives:

$$\begin{aligned}A^3 &= \left(125^{\frac{1}{3}}\right)^3 \\ &= 125^{\left(\frac{1}{3}\times3\right)} \\ &= 125^1 \\ &= 125\end{aligned}$$

Therefore, A is the number which multiplied 3 times by itself equals 125, that is 5. This expression is usually represented as "A is the 3rd-root of 125." In a more general form, if we have:

$$A = B^{\frac{1}{p}}$$

A is the number which multiplied p times by itself equals B, and we say that "*A is the pth-root of B.*"

Example Solve the equation:

$$64 = x^3$$

Solution: If we raise both sides to the power of $\frac{1}{3}$ (in other words, if we get the 3rd root of both sides), then:

$$\begin{aligned} 64^{\frac{1}{3}} &= \left(x^3\right)^{\frac{1}{3}} \\ &= x^{\left(3\times\frac{1}{3}\right)} \\ &= x^1 \\ &= x \end{aligned}$$

Therefore, x equals the 3rd-root of 64, which is 4 (because $4^3 = 64$).

In practical works, the numbers are not like those we have used in our examples; calculation with them is usually not easy without a calculator; and the answers are normally not exact; nonetheless, we can find the result with acceptable precision.

Example Lowe's formula for calculation of body surface area is:

$$S = 0.1 \times \text{wt}^{\frac{2}{3}}$$

where S represents the body surface area in m^2 and Wt is the body weight in kg. Calculate the body surface area of a girl weighing 20 kg.

Solution:

$$\begin{aligned} S &= 0.1 \times 20^{\frac{2}{3}} \\ &\approx 0.1 \times 7.37 \\ &\approx 0.737\text{m}^2 \end{aligned}$$

1.2 Logarithm

In the previous section, we have dealt with problems in which the base was unknown. Now, we want to solve problems with unknown powers, which are very important in practice.

Definition If

$$A = B^p$$

then, by definition, p is called the *logarithm* of A to the base B, and it is written as [1]:

$$p = \log_B A$$

Example If…

$$\begin{aligned}
&8 = 2^3 \quad \text{then} \quad 3 = \log_2 8 \\
&2 = 10^{0.301} \quad \text{then} \quad 0.301 = \log_{10} 2 \\
&\frac{1}{9} = 3^{-2} \quad \text{then} \quad -2 = \log_3 \frac{1}{9} \\
&M = 0.6^{9.1} \quad \text{then} \quad 9.1 = \log_{0.6} M
\end{aligned}$$

The most common types of logarithm which one commonly deals with in his or her work are those to base 10. These are called *common logarithms* in which the base is not usually written. Therefore, instead of writing $\log_{10}3$, it is common to write log 3.

Example The concentration of hydrogen ion (represented as $[H^+]$) in the most alkaline body fluid, the pancreatic juice, is about 0.000 000 03 mol/L. Express this value as a power of 10.

Solution: Mathematically, the problem is to solve the following equation:

$$0.00000003 = 10^x$$

Considering the definition of logarithm, we have

$$\begin{aligned}
x &= \log 0.000\ 000\ 03 \\
&= -7.523
\end{aligned}$$

Thus:

$$0.000000003 = 10^{-7.523}$$

Using our definition for logarithms, the following useful rules can be derived easily.

$$\log(A \times B) = \log A + \log B$$

Example

$$\begin{aligned}\log 300 &= \log(3 \times 100)\\ &= \log 3 + \log 100\\ &= 0.477 + 2\\ &= 2.477\end{aligned}$$

Example Suppose:

$$K = A \times B$$

calculate the $-\log K$.

Solution:

$$\begin{aligned}\log K &= \log(A \times B)\\ &= \log A + \log B\end{aligned}$$

and

$$\begin{aligned}-\log K &= -\left[\log(A \times B)\right]\\ &= -\log A - \log B\end{aligned}$$

*****

$$\log\left(\frac{A}{B}\right) = \log A - \log B$$

Example

$$\begin{aligned}\log 0.03 &= \log\left(\frac{3}{100}\right)\\ &= \log 3 - \log 100\\ &= 0.477 - 2\\ &= -1.523\end{aligned}$$

Example Assume:

$$K = \frac{A \times B}{C}$$

Then:

$$\begin{aligned}\log K &= \log\left(\frac{A \times B}{C}\right)\\ &= \log\left(A \times \frac{B}{C}\right)\\ &= \log A + \log\left(\frac{B}{C}\right)\\ &= \log A + \log B - \log C\end{aligned}$$

*****

$$\log 1 = 0$$

$$\log\left(\frac{1}{A}\right) = -\log A$$

Example

$$\log\frac{1}{\left[H^+\right]} = -\log\left[H^+\right]$$

where [H^+] represents the concentration of hydrogen ion. As an example, the [H^+] in pancreatic juice is about 0.000 000 03 mol/L, thus

$$\log\frac{1}{0.000\ 000\ 03} = -\log\left(0.000\ 000\ 03\right)$$
$$= 7.523$$

§§§§§

1.3 Chemical Equilibrium

Chemical reactions can either be reversible or irreversible. In reversible chemical reactions, an equilibrium state between the reactants and the product will be reached under certain circumstances of concentrations and temperature. An example is the dissociation of carbonic acid (H_2CO_3) to water (H_2O) and carbon dioxide (CO_2):

$$H_2CO_3 \rightarrow H_2O + CO_2 \tag{1.1}$$

Under a condition where the produced carbon dioxide can be swept away, complete conversion of carbonic acid to water and carbon dioxide is expected. On the other hand, if the pressure of CO_2 is high enough, it can react with water to form carbonic acid, according to the following reaction:

$$H_2O + CO_2 \rightarrow H_2CO_3 \tag{1.2}$$

This reaction is clearly the reverse of reaction (1.1). The fact that reactions (1.1) and (1.2) are reversible is represented by the following formulation:

$$H_2CO_3 \rightleftharpoons H_2O + CO_2 \tag{1.3}$$

When pure H_2CO_3 is in a closed container, it dissociates according to reaction (1.1). As CO_2 accumulates, its pressure increases and reaction (1.2) begins to occur at a higher rate which is accelerated as the pressure of CO_2 increases. Eventually, the rates of the decomposition reaction (1.1) and its reverse (1.2) reaction become equal, the pressure of CO_2 remains constant, and the system reaches an *equilibrium state*.

It is important to bear in mind that *the equilibrium state is dynamic*, i.e., by saying that the system of the reaction (1.3) reaches an equilibrium, it is not meant that the reaction is stopped completely; it means that the rate of decomposition of H_2CO_3 to H_2O and CO_2 equals the rate of formation of H_2CO_3 from H_2O and CO_2. Therefore, although no change occurs in the concentrations of reactants and products, the reaction continues.

If any of the factors that determine the equilibrium state of a system are changed, the system will respond in such a way to minimize the effect of the disturbance or the stress exerted. This is known as Le Chatelier's principle [2].

For example, by raising the pressure of CO_2 in the reaction (1.3), the rate of generation of H_2CO_3 overcomes its rate of dissociation. Therefore, the net reaction shifts to the left and more H_2CO_3 molecules are formed at the expense of the added CO_2. The externally applied stress (the increased pressure of CO_2) is reduced. At this point, the CO_2 pressure decreases (though it never reaches that of the previous equilibrium state), as it is used to form H_2CO_3; the decomposition of H_2CO_3 (from left to right) accelerates as more H_2CO_3 is produced. Ultimately, a new equilibrium state is reached where the rate of decomposition of H_2CO_3 equals the rate of its formation. The new concentration of H_2CO_3 is, however, higher than that it was in the previous equilibrium state.

On the other hand, if some H_2CO_3 is added to the system at equilibrium, the concentration of H_2CO_3 is increased; the rate of dissociation overcomes the rate of formation of H_2CO_3 and as a consequence, the externally increased H_2CO_3 concentration is diminished. The net reaction directs to the right and eventually, a new equilibrium state is reached.

Example Water ionizes according to the reversible reaction:

$$H_2O \rightleftharpoons H^+ + OH^-$$

What is the behavior of the system if…

(a) the concentration of H^+ is increased?
(b) the concentration of H^+ is decreased?

Solution: If the concentration of H^+ is increased, the Le Chatelier's principle predicts that the reaction proceeds in a direction to minimize the effect of this change, that is, a reaction which removes H^+ from the solution. The rate of formation of H_2O will be more than that of its dissociation; the reaction will thus shift to the left. On the contrary, by decreasing the concentration of H^+, the reaction will shift to the right to reach a new equilibrium state.

Example Carbonic acid ionizes according to the reversible reaction:

$$H_2CO_3 \rightleftharpoons HCO_3^- + H^+$$

Predict the behavior of the system if…
(a) the concentration of H^+ is increased.
(b) the concentration of H^+ is decreased.

Solution: As before, if you add some H^+ to the system, reconsidering the Le Chatelier's principle, the reaction proceeds in a way that removes the excess H^+ from the solution, that is, the formation of H_2CO_3 from H^+ and HCO_3^-. In the new equilibrium state, the concentration of H_2CO_3 will be increased relative to that in the initial state. According to the same discussion, reducing the concentration of H^+ will result in decreased H_2CO_3 concentration at the new equilibrium state.

1.3.1 Equilibrium Constant

Experiments reveal that, for a reaction of the form:

$$\alpha A + \beta B \rightleftharpoons \gamma C + \delta D$$

at equilibrium, the equilibrium constant (K) can be defined as:

$$K = \frac{[C]^{\gamma}[D]^{\delta}}{[A]^{\alpha}[B]^{\beta}}$$

where brackets ([]) represent the concentrations. This equilibrium constant only depends on the temperature of the reaction mixture.

Example For the ionization of water, we have:

$$H_2O \rightleftharpoons H^+ + OH^-$$

The equilibrium constant can then be written as:

$$K = \frac{[H^+][OH^-]}{[H_2O]}$$

For ionization of carbonic acid:

$$H_2CO_3 \rightleftharpoons HCO_3^- + H^+$$

the equilibrium constant is:

$$K = \frac{[HCO_3^-][H^+]}{[H_2O]}$$

Now, the basic concepts of mathematics and chemistry necessary for our following discussions have been reviewed, and we are ready to start understanding the "*Acid–Base Chemistry*."

1.4 Things to Remember

In general, for any A, B, C, p, and q we have

Powers

$$B^p \times B^q = B^{p+q}$$
$$\frac{B^p}{B^q} = B^{p-q}$$
$$B^0 = 1, \text{ if } B \neq 0$$
$$\left(B^p\right)^q = B^{p \times q}$$
$$B^{-p} = \frac{1}{B^p}$$
$$B^{\frac{1}{p}} = \sqrt[p]{B} \left(p^{th}\text{-root of } B\right)$$

Logarithm

$$\text{if } B \neq 0, \text{then} \ldots$$
$$A = B^C \Leftrightarrow C = \log_B A$$
$$\log_B \left(A \times C\right) = \log_B A + \log_B C$$
$$\log_B \frac{A}{C} = \log_B A - \log_B C$$
$$\log_B 1 = 0$$
$$\log_B \frac{1}{A} = -\log_B A$$
$$\log_B A^p = p \times \log_B A$$

§§§§§

Chemical Equilibrium

Le Chatelier's Principle
If any of the factors that determine the equilibrium state of a system are changed, the system will respond in such a way to minimize the effect of the disturbance or the stress exerted. This is known as Le Chatelier's principle.

Equilibrium Constant

For a reaction of the form:

$$\alpha A + \beta B \rightleftharpoons \gamma C + \delta D$$

at equilibrium, the equilibrium constant (K) is defined as:

$$K = \frac{[C]^{\gamma} [D]^{\delta}}{[A]^{\alpha} [B]^{\beta}}$$

References

1. Murray FJ. Logarithm. Encyclopædia Britannica; 2019. https://www.britannica.com/science/logarithm. Accessed 18 Nov 2020.
2. Russell JM. Simple models for teaching equilibrium and Le Châtelier's principle. J Chem Educ. 1988;65(10):871–2. https://doi.org/10.1021/ed065p871.

2 ABC's of Acid-Base Chemistry

2.1 Ionization of Water

Although water has only a very slight tendency to ionize, its products have intense biological effects [1]. Experiments indicate that water ionizes according to the reversible reaction:

$$H_2O \rightleftharpoons H^+ + OH^- \tag{2.1}$$

Using the general concepts of chemical equilibrium discussed in the previous chapter, for this reaction we can write:

$$K = \frac{\left[H^+\right]\left[OH^-\right]}{\left[H_2O\right]} \tag{2.2}$$

where K is the equilibrium constant, and $[H^+]$, $[OH^-]$, and $[H_2O]$ are concentrations of H^+, OH^-, and water, respectively. However, since the ionization is, at best, very small, the concentration of water in any aqueous solution is essentially constant and is equal to the number of grams of H_2O in 1 L, divided by the gram molecular weight, or 1000/18 = 55.5 mol/L; thus, it can be included in K and Eq. (2.2) can be written as:

$$K_w = K \times \left[H_2O\right] = \left[H^+\right]\left[OH^-\right] \tag{2.3}$$

K_w is called the *ion product of water*. It varies with temperature (Table 2.1). The ion product of water is 1×10^{-14} only at 25 °C; at other temperatures, the constant has different values.

F. Habibzadeh et al., *Pathophysiologic Basis of Acid-Base Disorders*,
https://doi.org/10.1007/978-981-16-0526-0_2

Table 2.1 Ion product of water, K_w and pK_w at a number of temperatures

Temperature (°C)	$K_w \times 10^{14}$	pK_w
0	0.114	14.943
10	0.292	14.535
25	1.008	13.997
40	2.919	13.535

2.2 *pH, pOH, pK, pK*$_w$

In the human body, the concentration of hydrogen ion ($[H^+]$) has a wide range. It is about 0.13 mol/L in the most acidic gastric juice, to about 0.000 000 03 mol/L in the most alkaline pancreatic juice. Working with these numbers is very difficult. However, they can be expressed as powers of 10 as follows:

$$0.13 = 10^{-0.886}$$

$$0.000\ 000\ 03 = 10^{-7.523}$$

Søren Peter Lauritz Sørensen, a Danish chemist, proposed the use of the *pH* (*p*uissance d'*H*ydrogen) scale to get rid of difficulties with expressing the concentration of hydrogen ion ($[H^+]$), which in normal biological settings usually involves negative exponents. The term *pH* is defined as the negative logarithm to the base 10 (common logarithm) of the hydrogen ion concentration ($[H^+]$) in solution [1, 2]. The definition can be written mathematically as:

$$pH = -\log\left[\mathrm{H}^+\right] \tag{2.4}$$

Similarly, the concentration of hydroxyl ion ($[OH^-]$) can be expressed on a *pOH* scale by the following definition:

$$pOH = -\log\left[\mathrm{OH}^-\right] \tag{2.5}$$

Example The concentrations of hydrogen ion and hydroxyl ion in the blood of a patient with a body temperature of 40 °C, are 4.02×10^{-8} and 7.26×10^{-7} mol/L, respectively. Calculate the corresponding *pH* and *pOH*.

Solution:

$$\left[\mathrm{H}^+\right] = 4.02 \times 10^{-8}\ \mathrm{mol/L}$$

By definition:

$$
\begin{aligned}
pH &= -\log\left[\mathrm{H}^+\right] \\
\text{then } pH &= -\log\left(4.02\times10^{-8}\right) \\
&= -\left(\log 4.02 + \log 10^{-8}\right) \\
&= -\left(0.604 - 8\right) \\
&= 7.396
\end{aligned}
$$

and

$$\left[\mathrm{OH}^-\right] = 7.26\times10^{-7}\ \mathrm{mol/L}$$

Thus:

$$
\begin{aligned}
pOH &= -\log\left[\mathrm{OH}^-\right] \\
\text{then } pOH &= -\log\left(7.26\times10^{-7}\right) \\
&= -\left(\log 7.26 + \log 10^{-7}\right) \\
&= -\left(0.861 - 7\right) \\
&= 6.139
\end{aligned}
$$

Now let's define pK and pK_w in the same way as follows:

$$pK = -\log K \tag{2.6}$$

and

$$pK_w = -\log K_w \tag{2.7}$$

For convention, in all of the previously defined terms (i.e., pH, pOH, pK, and pK_w), the symbol p denotes "*negative logarithm of…*"

Considering Eq. (2.3), we have:

$$K_w = \left[\mathrm{H}^+\right]\left[\mathrm{OH}^-\right]$$

where K_w is the ion product of water. Taking logarithm from both sides gives:

$$
\begin{aligned}
\log K_w &= \log\left(\left[\mathrm{H}^+\right]\left[\mathrm{OH}^-\right]\right) \\
&= \log\left[\mathrm{H}^+\right] + \log\left[\mathrm{OH}^-\right]
\end{aligned}
$$

Multiplying both sides by -1 yields:

$$-\log K_w = -\log\left[\mathrm{H}^+\right] + \left(-\log\left[\mathrm{OH}^-\right]\right)$$

employing Eqs. (2.4), (2.5), and (2.7), then:

$$pK_w = pH + pOH \tag{2.8}$$

The ion product of water (K_w) is 1×10^{-14} only at 25 °C, and consequently pK_w is 14 only at 25 °C; at other temperatures, it has other values [1]. Table 2.1 shows the values of K_w, and their corresponding pK_w at various temperatures.

Example Use the results of the previous example to confirm the Eq. (2.8).

Solution: In the previous example, our calculations showed that, $pH = 7.396$, and $pOH = 6.139$ at the body temperature of 40 °C. Then:

$$\begin{aligned} pH + pOH &= 7.396 + 6.139 \\ &= 13.535 \end{aligned}$$

which is the same as the value of pK_w at 40 °C (Table 2.1).

Example The pOH of a blood sample stored at 10 °C is measured at 7.520. What are the pH, and the hydrogen ion concentration in this sample?

Solution: Calling Table 2.1, the pK_w at 10 °C is 14.535. Using Eq. (2.8), we have:

$$\begin{aligned} pK_w &= pH + pOH \\ \text{then } pH &= pK_w - pOH \\ &= 14.535 - 7.520 \\ &= 7.015 \end{aligned}$$

By definition:

$$pH = -\log\left[\mathrm{H}^+\right]$$

Therefore:

$$\log\left[\mathrm{H}^+\right] = -pH$$

but, from the definition of logarithm:

$$\left[\mathrm{H}^+\right] = 10^{-pH}$$

and

$$\begin{aligned} \left[\mathrm{H}^+\right] &= 10^{-7.015} \\ &= 9.661 \times 10^{-8}\ \mathrm{mol/L} \\ &\approx 97\ \mathrm{nmol/L} \end{aligned}$$

Example At 37 °C, the extreme limits of hydrogen ion concentrations of arterial blood are 1.26×10^{-7} and 1.6×10^{-8} mol/L. What are the corresponding pH limits?

Solution: By definition:

$$pH = -\log\left[H^+\right]$$

Then:

$$\begin{aligned} pH_{min} &= -\log\left(1.26\times10^{-7}\right) \\ &= -\left(\log 1.26 + \log 10^{-7}\right) \\ &= 6.90\left(\text{Minimum}\right) \end{aligned}$$

and

$$\begin{aligned} pH_{max} &= -\log\left(1.68\times10^{-8}\right) \\ &= -\left(\log 1.68 + \log 10^{-8}\right) \\ &= 7.78\left(\text{Maximum}\right) \end{aligned}$$

Example The normal arterial blood *pH* is 7.4. Calculate the effect of…

(a) an increase of 2×10^{-8} mol/L in $[H^+]$,
(b) a decrement of 2×10^{-8} mol/L (the same quantity) in $[H^+]$.

Solution:

$$pH = -\log\left[H^+\right]$$

Then:

$$\begin{aligned} \left[H^+\right] &= 10^{-pH} \\ &= 10^{-7.4} \\ &= 4\times10^{-8}\ \text{mol/L} \\ &= 40\ \text{nmol/L} \end{aligned}$$

An increase of 2×10^{-8} mol/L in $[H^+]$ makes $[H^+]$ equal to 6×10^{-8} ($= 4 \times 10^{-8} + 2 \times 10^{-8}$) mol/L. Therefore, the corresponding *pH* is:

$$\begin{aligned} pH &= -\log\left[H^+\right] \\ &= -\log\left(6\times10^{-8}\right) \\ &= -\left(\log 6 + \log 10^{-8}\right) \\ &= 7.22 \end{aligned}$$

On the other hand, a decrease of 2×10^{-8} mol/L in $[H^+]$ makes $[H^+]$ equal to 2×10^{-8} $(= 4 \times 10^{-8} - 2 \times 10^{-8})$ mol/L, and the corresponding *pH* is:

$$\begin{aligned} pH &= -\log\left[H^+\right] \\ &= -\log\left(2 \times 10^{-8}\right) \\ &= -\left(\log 2 + \log 10^{-8}\right) \\ &= 7.70 \end{aligned}$$

Example Solve the previous example, if the original *pH* is 7.0 (instead of 7.4).

Solution: The solution is the same as before. It can easily be calculated that an increase of 2×10^{-8} mol/L in hydrogen ion concentration decreases the *pH* from 7.0 to 6.92. On the contrary, a decrease of 2×10^{-8} mol/L in hydrogen ion concentration increases the *pH* from 7.0 to 7.1.

As the two previous examples show, an equal change in the hydrogen ion concentration causes different changes in the *pH* scale, which depend on the original *pH*. It is also clear that the increase or decrease of hydrogen ions concentration causes unequal changes in *pH* (with the same original *pH*). Thereby, *the pH scale is not linear*, which means that equal intervals on the *pH* scale do not correspond to equal intervals on the hydrogen ion concentration scale.

Example The same volumes of two blood samples, having *pH* values of 7.2 and 7.6, respectively, are intermixed. What is the resultant *pH* in the final mixture?

Solution: The concentration of hydrogen ion in the first blood sample is:

$$\begin{aligned} \left[H^+\right]_1 &= 10^{-pH_1} \\ &= 10^{-7.2} \\ &= 6.31 \times 10^{-8} \text{ mol/L} \end{aligned}$$

and in the second sample, it can be calculated to be:

$$\begin{aligned} \left[H^+\right]_2 &= 10^{-pH_2} \\ &= 10^{-7.6} \\ &= 2.51 \times 10^{-8} \text{ mol/L} \end{aligned}$$

The volumes of the samples are the same, thus the hydrogen ion concentration of the resultant mixture will be:

$$\left[H^+\right]_{\text{final}} = \frac{\left[H^+\right]_1 + \left[H^+\right]_2}{2} = \frac{6.31\times10^{-8} + 2.51\times10^{-8}}{2} = 4.41\times10^{-8}\ \text{mol/L}$$

Then:

$$pH_{\text{final}} = -\log\left[H^+\right]_{\text{final}} = -\log\left(4.41\times10^{-8}\right) = 7.36$$

Note that the mean value of pH_1 and pH_2 is:

$$pH_{\text{mean}} = \frac{pH_1 + pH_2}{2} = \frac{7.2 + 7.6}{2} = 7.4$$

which is different from the actual calculated value of 7.36. So *it is not correct to take arithmetical means of pH values*; instead, the individual *pH* values should be converted to their corresponding hydrogen ion concentration; the resultant hydrogen ion concentration must then be calculated; and finally, this value must be reconverted to its corresponding *pH*.

2.3 Acids and Bases

Acids and bases influence many biological activities, and equilibria involving them are perhaps one of the major classes of equilibria.

Historically, acids were recognized by their sour taste (from Latin *acidus* meaning sour; *acetum*, vinegar); alkalis (from Arabic *al kali* meaning ashes of a plant) were considered those substances that could neutralize the effects of acids. The chemical properties of acids are the results of their reversible dissociation into ions, one of which is H^+.

In 1923, Lowry and Brønsted proposed their general concept of acids and bases [3]. According to the Lowry-Brønsted definition, *an acid is a substance that has a tendency to donate a proton* (H^+), whereas *a base has the tendency to accept a proton*. Carbonic acid (H_2CO_3) ionizes according to this reversible reaction:

H_2CO_3	$\rightleftharpoons$	$H_2CO_3^-$	+	H^+
Proton donor		Proton acceptor		Proton

Using the Lowry-Brønsted concept, carbonic acid (H_2CO_3) is an acid because it donates H^+ and bicarbonate ion (HCO_3^-) is a base because it accepts H^+. A proton donor (acid) and its corresponding proton acceptor (base) make up a *conjugate acid-base pair*. Another example is the ammonium (NH_4^+)-ammonia (NH_3) conjugate acid-base pair. Ammonium ion (NH_4^+) dissociates according to the reversible reaction:

NH_4^+	$\rightleftharpoons$	NH_3	+	H^+
Proton donor, conjugate acid		Proton acceptor, conjugate base		Proton

Using the general definition, NH_4^+ is an acid, and NH_3 is its conjugate base.

In the same way, the ionization of acetic acid can be written as:

CH_3COOH	$\rightleftharpoons$	CH_3COO^-	+	H^+
Proton donor, conjugate acid		Proton acceptor, conjugate base		Proton

There are many conjugate acid-base pairs in the body, some of which will be discussed later in more detail.

Now, let us apply the concepts of equilibrium constant to the equilibrium involving conjugate acid-base pairs. Carbonic acid dissociates according to the reaction:

H_2CO_3	$\rightleftharpoons$	$H_2CO_3^-$	+	H^+
Proton donor, conjugate acid		Proton acceptor, conjugate base		Proton

The equilibrium constant of this reaction is:

$$K_1 = \frac{[H^+][HCO_3^-]}{[H_2CO_3]} = [H^+]\cdot\frac{[HCO_3^-]}{[H_2CO_3]} \tag{2.9}$$

The concentration of carbonic acid in a solution is proportional to the concentration of dissolved carbon dioxide [CO_2], thus Eq. (2.9) becomes:

$$K_1 = [H^+]\cdot\frac{[HCO_3^-]}{K_2[CO_2]}$$

Therefore:

$$K_1K_2 = [H^+]\cdot\frac{[HCO_3^-]}{[CO_2]} \tag{2.10}$$

Both K_1 and K_2 are constants and, consequently, their multiplication is also a constant, namely K, which equals:

$$K = \left[\mathrm{H}^+\right] \cdot \frac{\left[\mathrm{HCO}_3^-\right]}{\left[\mathrm{CO}_2\right]}$$

Taking the logarithm of both sides gives:

$$\log K = \log\left[\mathrm{H}^+\right] + \log\frac{\left[\mathrm{HCO}_3^-\right]}{\left[\mathrm{CO}_2\right]}$$

rearranging the terms, then:

$$-\log\left[\mathrm{H}^+\right] = -\log K + \log\frac{\left[\mathrm{HCO}_3^-\right]}{\left[\mathrm{CO}_2\right]} \tag{2.11}$$

Considering Eqs. (2.4) and (2.6), Eq. (2.11) can be rewritten as:

$$pH = pK + \log\frac{\left[\mathrm{HCO}_3^-\right]}{\left[\mathrm{CO}_2\right]} \tag{2.12}$$

which is known as the *Henderson-Hasselbalch equation*, which can be stated in a more general form as:

$$pH = pK + \log\frac{\left[\text{Proton acceptor}\right]}{\left[\text{Proton donor}\right]} \tag{2.13}$$

Example In a normal healthy person, the quotient of $\left[\mathrm{HCO}_3^-\right]$ to the concentration of dissolved CO_2 is about 20. If the normal arterial pH is 7.4 at the body temperature of 37 °C, calculate the value of pK for this system in the body.

Solution: Henderson-Hasselbalch equation for this system (Eq. (2.12)) states that:

$$pH = pK + \log\frac{\left[\mathrm{HCO}_3^-\right]}{\left[\mathrm{CO}_2\right]}$$

inserting the known values and solving for pK, we have:

$$\begin{aligned} pK &= pH - \log\frac{\left[\mathrm{HCO}_3^-\right]}{\left[\mathrm{CO}_2\right]} \\ &= 7.4 - \log 20 \\ &= 7.4 - 1.3 \\ &= 6.1 \end{aligned}$$

Example The pH of an arterial blood sample from a patient with chronic renal failure (CRF) is 7.2. If the concentration of the bicarbonate ion ($\left[HCO_3^-\right]$) is 6.07 mmol/L, calculate the concentration of the dissolved CO_2 ($[CO_2]$).

Solution: As the Henderson-Hasselbalch equation states:

$$pH = pK + \log\frac{\left[HCO_3^-\right]}{\left[CO_2\right]}$$

from the previous example, the value of pK at 37 °C is 6.1. Inserting the known values in the equation, then:

$$7.2 = 6.1 + \log\frac{6.07}{\left[CO_2\right]}$$

Solving for $[CO_2]$, we have

$$\log\frac{6.07}{\left[CO_2\right]} = 7.2 - 6.1$$
$$= 1.1$$

Then:

$$\frac{6.07}{\left[CO_2\right]} = 10^{1.1}$$
$$= 12.59$$

Thus:

$$\left[CO_2\right] = \frac{6.07}{12.59}$$
$$= 0.48\,\text{mmol} / \text{L}$$

Equilibrium constants for ionization reactions, like those of the dissociation of acids and bases, are more usually called *ionization* or *dissociation constants.*

Table 2.2 The dissociation constant and corresponding pK of some common acids, measured at 25 °C

Acid (proton donor)	K	pK
CH_3COOH (acetic acid)	1.74×10^{-5}	4.76
$CH_3CHOHCOOH$ (lactic acid)	1.38×10^{-4}	3.86
H_3PO_4 (phosphoric acid)	7.25×10^{-3}	2.14
$H_2PO_4^-$ (dihydrogen phosphate ion)	1.38×10^{-7}	6.86
H_2CO_3 (carbonic acid)	1.70×10^{-4}	3.77
NH_4^+ (ammonium ion)	5.60×10^{-10}	9.25

Acids have different tendencies to donate a proton. The stronger acids, such as hydrochloric acid (HCl), have higher dissociation constants (and consequently, lower *pK*); weaker acids, such as carbonic acid (H_2CO_3), have lower dissociation constants (higher *pK*). Table 2.2 shows the values of dissociation constant of a number of acids and their corresponding *pK* values measured at 25 °C.

Many biological activities and most of the biological reactions depend on the $[H^+]/[OH^-]$ ratio. Normal conformation and the charge state of proteins, which play an important role in their normal structure and function, depend on a stable invariant and usually a neutral electrochemical environment [4]. In most cases, a neutral intracellular environment is provided, in which the concentration of hydrogen ion ($[H^+]$) and hydroxyl ion ($[OH^-]$) are equal, thus a constant ratio $[H^+]/[OH^-]$ of 1 is maintained, which preserves the normal charge state of cytosolic metabolites, and in effect, maintains active sites of intracellular enzymes.

Example The pK_w at 25 °C is 14. What is the neutral *pH* at this temperature?

Solution: By definition, the neutral state is achieved when the ratio $[H^+]/[OH^-]$ equals to 1, thus:

$$\left[H^+\right]=\left[OH^-\right]$$

taking negative logarithm of both sides gives:

$$-\log\left[H^+\right]=-\log\left[OH^-\right]$$

substituting *pH*, and *pOH* for $-\log[H^+]$, and $-\log[OH^-]$, respectively, then:

$$pH = pOH$$

but from Eq. (2.8), we have:

$$pK_w = pH + pOH$$

Therefore, in a neutral state we have:

$$\begin{aligned} pH = pOH &= \frac{pK_w}{2} \\ &= \frac{14}{2} \\ &= 7 \end{aligned}$$

As a result, using a pK_w of 13.7 at 37 °C (normal body temperature), *the pH of neutral intracellular milieu should be around 6.85* (= 13.7/2).

Example The normal blood and extracellular fluid *pH* is about 7.4. Determine the ratio of intracellular to extracellular hydrogen ion concentrations.

Solution: If $[H^+]_i$ and $[H^+]_e$ designate intracellular and extracellular hydrogen ion concentrations, respectively, then, assuming a neutral intracellular *milieu*, from the previous example, we have:

$$pH_i = -\log\left[H^+\right]_i = 6.85$$

Therefore:

$$\begin{aligned}\left[H^+\right]_i &= 10^{-6.85}\\ &= 1.41\times10^{-7}\ \text{mol/L}\end{aligned}$$

and

$$pH_e = -\log\left[H^+\right]_e = 7.4$$

Thus:

$$\begin{aligned}\left[H^+\right]_e &= 10^{-7.4}\\ &= 3.98\times10^{-8}\ \text{mol/L}\end{aligned}$$

Then:

$$\frac{\left[H^+\right]_i}{\left[H^+\right]_e} = \frac{1.41\times10^{-7}}{3.98\times10^{-8}} \approx 3.5$$

Therefore, the normal intracellular concentration of hydrogen ion is about 3–4 times greater than its extracellular concentration. This normal intracellular to extracellular hydrogen ion concentration gradient promotes unloading and the removal of cellular acidic waste products, including CO_2, from the cell to extracellular space and blood. This means that, *for neutrality of intracellular space, blood and extracellular fluid should be normally relatively alkaline*, and this is why the normal arterial blood *pH* is maintained in the range 7.35–7.45.

In severely diabetic patients, the *pH* of arterial blood is lower than 7.35. This condition is called *acidemia* (adding of an acid to a solution lowers the *pH*). In contrast, in some situations, the arterial blood *pH* is higher than 7.45, a condition called *alkalemia.*

Buffers can preserve intracellular and extracellular *pH* within a narrow range, but what is a buffer?

2.4 Buffers

Solutions composed of an acid-base conjugate pair (i.e., an acid and one of its salts, or a base and one of its salts), exhibit the ability to resist changes in *pH*, when some acid or base is added to them. Such solutions, having the property of preventing a change in their *pH* are called *buffer* solutions, or simply buffers [1]. In this respect, solutions composed of weak acid or base are more effective. Therefore, a mixture of carbonic acid (conjugate acid) and bicarbonate (conjugate base), ($H_2CO_3 + HCO_3^-$) is a buffer.

2.4.1 Buffering Action

The buffering ability is neither a miracle nor a matter of black magic! In a mixture composed of a weak acid *HA*, and one of its salts, the hydrogen ion concentration of the solution is determined by the dissociation constant of the acid (stronger acid produces higher hydrogen ion concentration and lower *pH*).

When hydrogen ions are added to this solution in the form of some acid, the equilibrium is disturbed by the presence of excess hydrogen ions, and the *pH* of the solution is lowered. As was mentioned earlier, this is a stress for the system and according to Le Chatelier's principle, the system behaves in such a way as to minimize the effect of disturbance. To remove these excess hydrogen ions and to re-establish the ionization equilibrium, hydrogen ions are combined with anions of salt A^- (conjugate base) to form molecules of unionized acid *HA* (conjugate acid). Therefore, the *pH* of the solution returns to a value near that of its original.

Again, when some base is added to the mixture of an acid and one of its salts, the excess of hydroxyl ions alters the equilibrium of water. To re-establish this equilibrium, hydrogen and hydroxyl ions combine to form water. As the latter reaction removes some hydrogen ions, it elevates the *pH* of the solution. However, removal of hydrogen ions from the mixture in turn perturbs the acid equilibrium. Considering Le Chatelier's principle, the system responds in such a way as to increase the hydrogen ion concentration and consequently lowers the *pH*. To re-establish the acid equilibrium, some of the acid *HA* (conjugate acid) ionizes to produce the requisite hydrogen ions. The net outcome of these reactions is that the excess hydroxyl ions are essentially neutralized, and the *pH* of the solution reverts to a *pH* close to its original value.

These considerations are employed when the quantity of the acid or base added to a buffer is not so much as to alter the ratio of conjugate base to conjugate acid to any great extent. The buffering action of a weak base *BOH* and one of its salts can be interpreted in the same way.

The maximum buffering capacity for a given buffer is when the pH of solution is equal to the pK of that system [1]. When the *pH* is lower than the *pK*, the buffer can stand excess hydroxyl better than hydrogen ions; if the *pH* is higher than the *pK*, excess hydrogen ions can be buffered better than excess hydroxyl ions.

One of the major buffers in extracellular fluid is phosphate. In this system, dihydrogen phosphate ion ($H_2PO_4^-$) acts as conjugate acid and is in equilibrium with monohydrogen phosphate ion (HPO_4^{2-}) which behaves as conjugate base, according to the reversible reaction:

$$H_2PO_4^- \rightleftharpoons HPO_4^{2-} + H^+$$

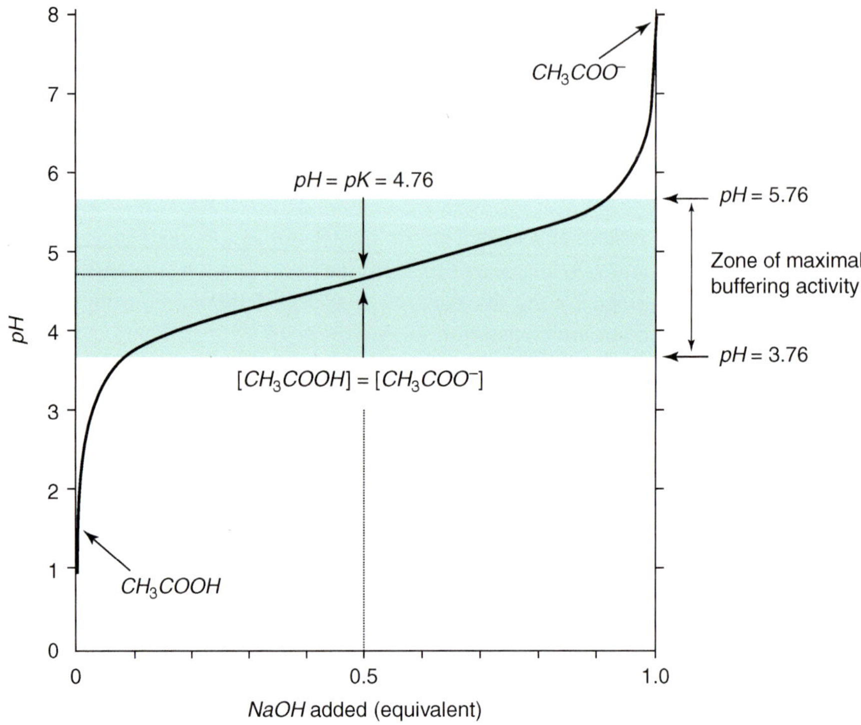

Fig. 2.1 Titration curve of acetic acid

The normal extracellular *pH* of 7.4 is a little higher than the *pK* of this reaction, which is 6.86 (Table 2.2). Therefore, this system can stand excess hydrogen ions (acidosis) better than excess hydroxyl ions (alkalosis).

2.4.2 Titration and Titration Curve

The quantity of an acid in a given solution can be found by titration that is adding some base with a known concentration to a known volume of acid solution to reach the neutral state. The base (usually NaOH) is added gradually until the acid is entirely neutralized, as detected with an indicator (e.g., phenolphthalein) or a *pH* meter. Then the concentration of the acid being titrated can be found simply. A plot of the *pH* of the solution under titration against the amount of added base to this point is called a *titration curve*. The titration curve of acetic acid, a typical weak acid, is shown in Fig. 2.1. If the titration of a 0.1 molar solution of acetic acid with 0.1 molar NaOH at 25 °C is traced, it can be seen that, in this process, the following reversible reactions are involved:

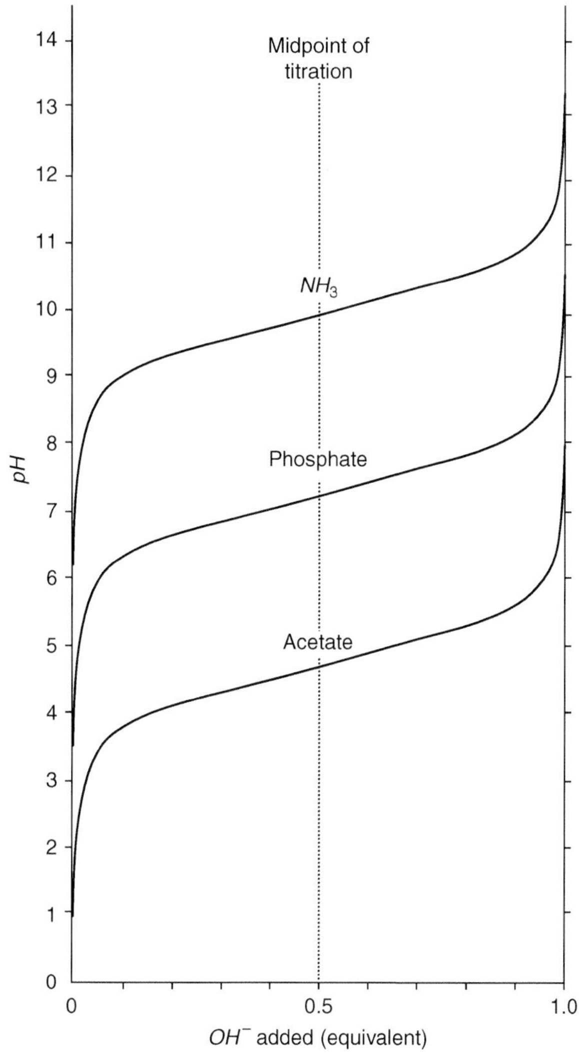

Fig. 2.2 Comparison of titration curves of three acids

$$H_2O \rightleftharpoons H^+ + OH^-$$
$$CH_3COOH \rightleftharpoons H^+ + CH_3COO^-$$

At the start of the titration (before adding NaOH), the acetic acid is slightly ionized. When successive increments of NaOH (hydroxyl ions, OH^-) are added to the solution, the excess hydroxyl ions combine with hydrogen ions (H^+) to form water and alter the equilibrium of water. As previously mentioned, the system reacts to this external stress in such a way as to minimize the disturbance, that is, the dissociation of unionized acetic acid to acetate and H^+. By adding more increments of base, this reaction will continue to a point at which there is no unionized acid molecule; this is the endpoint of the titration.

The titration can be reversed, starting from the neutralization point to the original state by the addition of H^+ to the solution, following the exact same path.

Referring to Fig. 2.1, a flattened zone around the *pH* 4.76, which equals the *pK* of acetic acid (Table 2.2), is seen. Around this flattened region, the addition or removal of base (OH^-) (or, the removal or addition of acid (H^+)) has a minimal effect on the solution *pH*. Therefore, the solution opposes any change in its *pH*. This point where the *pH* is equal to the *pK*, as was noted earlier, corresponds to the maximal buffering activity. At this point, the concentrations of conjugate base (CH_3COO^-), and the conjugate acid (CH_3COOH) are the same.

Different weak acids or bases have virtually the same titration curve in the shape, and their buffering activity correspond to a flattened area in their curves. For comparison, the titration curves of some acids are given in Fig. 2.2.

2.4.3 Amino Acids as Buffers

Substances with the carboxyl group (–COOH) can donate proton and therefore, by definition, are acids. They dissociate according to the reversible reaction:

$$\underset{\substack{\text{Proton donor}\\(\text{acid})}}{R-COOH} \rightleftharpoons R-COO^- + H^+$$

Acetic acid is an example of these substances.

Species with the *amino group* ($-NH_2$) can accept proton, and therefore are bases. The reaction is:

$$\underset{\substack{\text{Proton}\\\text{acceptor}\\(\text{base})}}{R-NH_2} + H^+ \rightleftharpoons R-NH_3^+$$

An *amino acid*, as its name implies, is an acid with the amino group. It can react as an acid or as a base, depending on the concentration of hydrogen ion. In low hydrogen ion concentration (high *pH*), it acts as an acid, according to the reversible reaction:

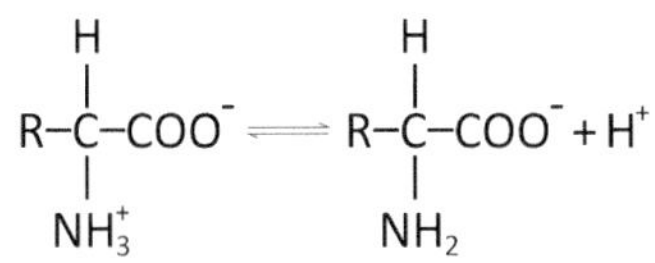

Pronton donor
(acid)

In high concentration of hydrogen ion (low *pH*), it behaves as a base:

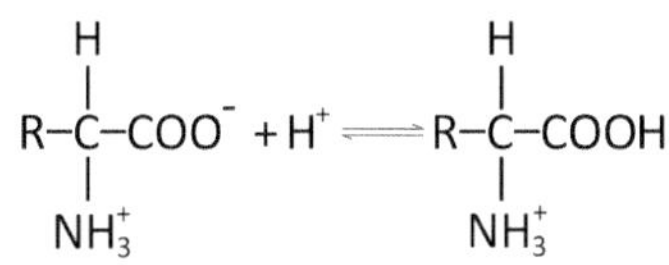

Pronton acceptor
(base)

Compounds having this two-way property (both acid and base) are *amphoteric* (from Greek *amphi* meaning both).

There are different chemical groups, including the amino group ($-NH_2$), the carboxyl group ($-COOH$), and the imidazole group (e.g., in amino acid histidine), which can donate or accept hydrogen ion under some conditions. Therefore, they can possess a buffering activity at some *pH*. Substances containing these chemical groups can thus act as buffers. *Proteins, which are made of amino acids, are the most important buffers in the cell.*

2.5 Things to Remember

pH, *pOH*, *pK*, and *pK*$_w$

For convention, the symbol *p* is defined as "negative logarithm of…," thus:

$$\begin{aligned} pH &= -\log\left[\mathrm{H}^+\right] \ (\text{as defined by S}\varnothing\text{rensen}) \\ pOH &= -\log\left[\mathrm{OH}^-\right] \\ pK &= -\log K \\ pK_w &= -\log K_w \end{aligned}$$

and we have

$$pK_w = p\mathrm{H} + p\mathrm{OH}$$

Equal changes in the hydrogen ion concentration cause unequal changes in *pH*, which depend on the original *pH*. The *pH* scale is not linear.

Acid and Base

Lowry-Brønsted Definition

An acid is a substance that has a tendency to donate a proton (H^+), whereas a base has the tendency to accept a proton. Acids have different tendencies to donate a proton. Stronger acids have higher dissociation constants (lower *pK*), whereas weaker acids have lower dissociation constants (higher *pK*).

The *pH* of intracellular space is around 6.85 (neutral *pH*). For maintaining the intracellular neutrality, blood and extracellular fluid should normally be relatively alkaline, and this is why the normal arterial blood *pH* is preserved between 7.35 and 7.45.

Buffers

Buffers can preserve intracellular and extracellular *pH* within a narrow range. Solutions composed of an acid-base conjugate pair possess the ability to resist changes in *pH*, when some acid or base is added to them. Such solutions, having the property of preventing a change in their *pH*, are called buffers. The maximum buffering capacity for a given buffer is when the *pH* of solution is equal to the *pK* of that system. Proteins are the most important buffers in the cell.

References

1. Nelson DL, Lehninger AL, Cox MM. Lehninger principles of biochemistry. New York: W.H. Freeman; 2008.
2. Severinghaus JW, Astrup PB. History of blood gas analysis. I. The development of electrochemistry. J Clin Monit. 1985;1(3):180–92. https://doi.org/10.1007/BF02832259.
3. Kauffrnan GB. The Bronsted-Lowry acid base concept. J Chem Educ. 1988;65(1):28–31. https://doi.org/10.1021/ed065p28.
4. Rahn H, Reeves RB, Howell BJ. Hydrogen ion regulation, temperature, and evolution. Am Rev Respir Dis. 1975;112(2):165–72. https://doi.org/10.1164/arrd.1975.112.2.165.

Gas Laws

3

3.1 Pressure and Partial Pressure of a Gas

The pressure of a gas is a measure of the molecular bombardment on the walls of its container. In the same way, the pressure in a gaseous mixture is the result of the molecular motion in its container. The amount of pressure each gas applies depends on its own number of molecules. The greater the number of molecules which hit each unit area, the greater the pressure applied. Therefore, in a mixture of gases the pressure each gas exerts depends on temperature (i.e., their energy), and the ratio of its number of molecules to the total number of molecules in the container, which is the mole fraction. In a gaseous mixture, the pressure each gas exerts is called *partial pressure* and we can write:

$$p_i = \frac{n_i}{n} p \tag{3.1}$$

where p_i and n_i denote partial pressure and number of moles of the ith gas, respectively. p is the total pressure and n is the number of moles of gases in the container. An equal number of moles of any gas occupies the same volume. Therefore, the fraction of a gas by volume is equal to its mole fraction. Thus, Eq. (3.1) can be rewritten as:

$$p_i = \frac{v_i}{v} p$$

where v_i and v are volume of the ith gas and the total volume of the gaseous mixture, respectively. Then:

$$p_i = f_i \times p \tag{3.2}$$

where f_i designates the fractional volume of the ith gas.

F. Habibzadeh et al., *Pathophysiologic Basis of Acid-Base Disorders*,
https://doi.org/10.1007/978-981-16-0526-0_3

Example At sea level, dry air composes of 20.93% oxygen, 0.03% carbon dioxide, and 79.04% nitrogen. Calculate the partial pressure of each gas.

Solution: At sea level, the total pressure of the gaseous mixture (barometric pressure) is 760 mm Hg. The above values are the fractional volumes of the gases in the air. Using Eq. (3.2), we have:

$$
\begin{aligned}
pO_2 &= \frac{20.93}{100} \times 760 \\
&= 159.07\,\text{mm Hg} \\
pCO_2 &= \frac{0.03}{100} \times 760 \\
&= 0.23\,\text{mm Hg} \\
pN_2 &= \frac{79.04}{100} \times 760 \\
&= 600.70\,\text{mm Hg}
\end{aligned}
$$

3.2 Dalton's Law of Partial Pressure

Different gases introduced into the same container mix rapidly. Dalton's law of partial pressure states that at constant temperature the total pressure applied by a mixture of gases in a certain volume is equal to the sum of the individual pressure (partial pressure) which each gas would exert if it occupied the same total volume alone [1].

Example Considering the results of the previous example, try to check the Dalton's law of partial pressure.

Solution: As you have seen, the partial pressures of oxygen, carbon dioxide, and nitrogen in dry air and at sea level (p = 760 mm Hg), are 159.07, 0.23, and 600.70 mm Hg, respectively. Dalton's law states that the sum of the partial pressures must be equal to the total pressure of 760 mm Hg:

$$159.07 + 0.23 + 600.70 = 760\,\text{mm Hg}$$

which is correct.

3.3 Composition of Alveolar Air

The gas mixture in the alveolar space is called alveolar air. Alveolar air is composed of oxygen, carbon dioxide, and nitrogen. Water vapor also exists in the alveolar air. This water has been vaporized from the surface of the respiratory tract [1]. Like any other gas, water vapor also applies a pressure, but alveolar air is saturated with water, meaning that the number of water molecules exiting the mucosal surface is exactly equal to the number of molecules re-entering. As a result, the number of water molecules cannot be further increased. Therefore, the *saturated water vapor pressure* is only a function of temperature, and at normal body temperature of 37 °C is 47 mm Hg [2].

The alveolar air pressure is exactly equal to the atmospheric pressure (760 mm Hg at sea level). Employing Dalton's law, we have:

$$p_{\text{Alveolar air}} = p_{\text{Alveolar dry air}} + p_{\text{Water vapor}}$$

Substituting 47 mm Hg for saturated water vapor pressure at 37 °C, it becomes:

$$p_{\text{B}} = p_{\text{Alveolar dry air}} + 47$$

where p_{B} is the barometric (atmospheric) pressure. Then:

$$p_{\text{Alveolar dry air}} = p_{\text{B}} - 47$$

Example Calculate the partial pressure of nitrogen in the alveolar space, when the barometric pressure is 740 mm Hg, and the inspired air contains 79% nitrogen, in a normal person.

Solution: Inspired air passes through the airways and is humidified. When it reaches the alveolar space, it is fully saturated with water, but its total pressure is exactly equal to the barometric pressure. The nitrogen content of the dry part of the alveolar air is exactly similar to the inspired air (because there is no net nitrogen exchange). Therefore, if inspired air contains 79% nitrogen, the dry part of the alveolar air also contains the same fraction. In a normal person with a body temperature of 37 °C, we have:

$$\begin{aligned} p_{\text{Alveolar dry air}} &= p_{\text{B}} - 47\,\text{mm Hg} \\ &= 740 - 47\,\text{mm Hg} \\ &= 693\,\text{mm Hg} \end{aligned}$$

and

$$p\text{N}_2 = f_i\text{N}_2 \times p$$

Therefore:

$$\begin{aligned} p\text{N}_2 &= \frac{79}{100} \times 693 \\ &= 547.5\,\text{mm Hg} \end{aligned}$$

3.4 Gas-Liquid Equilibrium

Gases dissolve in liquids. When a gas is in contact with a liquid, the molecules of the gas in their continuous motion impinge on the surface of the liquid. Some mix with the molecules of the liquid, and are said to be dissolved. At any given temperature and pressure, a gas dissolves in a given liquid only to a certain degree. When the rate of diffusion of the gas into the solution is counterbalanced by the rate of diffusion out, the system reaches a state of equilibrium between the gas over the liquid and the gas dissolved in it.

It is a convention to state that the gas in solution exerts the same *tension* (or *partial pressure*) as the partial pressure of the gas over the liquid in equilibrium with it. This definition of tension (or partial pressure) of a dissolved gas offers the clue to a method whereby the tension (partial pressure) of a gas (say oxygen) in a liquid (say blood) can be measured. A small amount of the blood is brought into contact with samples of oxygen at varying known pressures, until one is found where oxygen neither enters nor leaves the blood. The oxygen in the blood has the same tension as the partial pressure of the sample of oxygen with which it is in contact. Although this method is easy to understand, it is not used in practice. In modern analyzers, partial pressures of different gases are measured by means of specially designed blood gas electrodes.

Example An arterial blood sample is *wrongly* transferred to the blood gas analyzer in direct contact with the ambient air. Calculate the pO_2 (partial pressure of oxygen) of this sample, if the barometric pressure is 640 mm Hg.

Solution: During the sample transferal, the oxygen in the air equilibrates with the dissolved oxygen in the blood. Regarding the oxygen fractional concentration of 21% in the air, then:

$$\begin{aligned} pO_2 &= f_iO_2 \times p_B \\ &= \frac{21}{100} \times 640 \\ &= 134.4\,\text{mm Hg} \end{aligned}$$

This value obviously does not reflect the arterial oxygen tension of the patient. The same discussion is true for the partial pressures of all other gases in this sample (e.g., CO_2, N_2), and this is why *the blood sample for gas analysis must be transferred by an air-tight vessel.*

3.5 Henry's Law

Henry's law states that the amount of a given gas (e.g., CO_2) which dissolves in a liquid (e.g., blood) is directly proportional to the partial pressure of the gas. Thus, for any gas we have:

$$C = \alpha\, p \tag{3.3}$$

where C designates the concentration of gas in liquid (in mL of gas per 100 mL), p denotes the gas tension (in mm Hg), and α is the proportionality constant, the so-called *solubility constant*. The value of α (solubility constant) for dissolved carbon dioxide in blood is 0.0301 mmol/L per mm Hg at a temperature of 38 °C [3], therefore:

$$[CO_2] = 0.0301\, pCO_2 \tag{3.4}$$

$[CO_2]$ denotes CO_2 concentration in mmol/L, and pCO_2 is the partial pressure of carbon dioxide in blood in mm Hg.

Example The normal value for $[CO_2]$ in arterial blood is 1.2 mmol/L. What is the normal arterial pCO_2 (partial pressure of arterial CO_2)?

Solution:

$$[CO_2] = \alpha\, pCO_2$$
$$1.2 = 0.0301\, pCO_2$$

Therefore:

$$pCO_2 = \frac{1.2}{0.0301} \approx 40\,\text{mm Hg}$$

Example What is the normal concentration of bicarbonate ($[HCO_3^-]$) in arterial blood?

Solution: Recalling Henderson-Hasselbalch equation (Eq. (2.12)):

$$pH = pK + \log\frac{[HCO_3^-]}{[CO_2]} \tag{2.12}$$

and replacing the known normal values, we have:

$$7.4 = 6.1 + \log\frac{[HCO_3^-]}{1.2}$$

solving for $[HCO_3^-]$, then:

$$[HCO_3^-] = 1.2 \times 10^{(7.4-6.1)} \approx 24\,\text{mmol / L}$$

In acid-base problems, it is more usual to use the partial pressure than the concentration of CO_2. Substituting $\alpha\, pCO_2$ for $[CO_2]$ in Eq. (2.12) gives:

$$pH = pK + \log\frac{[HCO_3^-]}{\alpha\, pCO_2} \tag{3.5}$$

Example A 6-year-old girl is brought to the emergency room (ER) with barbiturate poisoning. Her respiration is shallow, with a rate of 10 breaths per minute. The measured arterial pCO_2 is 52 mm Hg, and the concentration of bicarbonate in her arterial blood is 25.5 mmol/L. Determine the arterial *pH*.

Solution: Using Eq. (3.5), then:

$$\begin{aligned} pH &= pK + \log\frac{\left[HCO_3^-\right]}{\alpha\, pCO_2} \\ &= 6.1 + \log\frac{25.5}{0.0301 \times 52} \\ &= 7.31 \end{aligned}$$

The *pH* is lower than normal (7.35–7.45). Therefore, the patient has acidemia.

Solution of oxygen, like any gas, in a liquid also obeys Henry's law, that is, the amount of dissolved O_2 is proportional to the pO_2 (partial pressure of oxygen) [1]. Therefore, we can write:

$$vO_2 = s\, pO_2 \tag{3.6}$$

where vO_2 is the volume of oxygen dissolved in 100 mL of solution (e.g., blood), and *s* is the *solubility coefficient* of oxygen and its numerical value for blood is 0.003 mL/100 mL of blood per mm Hg of oxygen, at a temperature of 38 °C [4]. This means that, at 38 °C, under an oxygen pressure of 1 mm Hg, there are 0.003 mL dissolved oxygen in 100 mL of blood. When the partial pressure of oxygen differs from 1 mm Hg, the amount of dissolved oxygen is proportionally different.

Example The partial pressure of oxygen in an arterial blood sample is 110 mm Hg. What is the amount of dissolved O_2 in this sample, if the temperature is 38 °C?

Solution: We have:

$$\begin{aligned} vO_2 &= s\, pO_2 \\ &= 0.003 \times 110 \\ &= 0.33\,\text{mL } O_2/100 \text{ mL blood} \end{aligned}$$

To this point, you have learned the basic concepts of acid-base chemistry and blood gases. In the next chapter, you will see what happens in a normal person.

3.6 Things to Remember

Partial Pressure of Gases

In a gaseous mixture, the pressure each gas exerts is called partial pressure and we can write:

$$p_i = f_i\, p$$

where p, p_i, and f_i denote total gas pressure, partial pressure, and fractional volume of the ith gas, respectively.

It is a convention to state that the gas in solution exerts the same tension (or partial pressure) as the partial pressure of the gas over the liquid in equilibrium with it.

Dalton's Law of Partial Pressure

At constant temperature, the total pressure applied by a mixture of gases in a certain volume is equal to the sum of the individual pressure which each gas would exert if it occupied the same total volume alone.

Alveolar Air

The gas mixture in the alveolar space is called alveolar air and:

$$p_{\text{Alveolar dry air}} = p_{\text{B}} - 47$$

where p_{B} is the barometric (atmospheric) pressure.

Henry's Law

The amount of a given gas which dissolves in a liquid is directly proportional to the partial pressure of gas. Therefore:

$$[CO_2] = 0.0301\, pCO_2$$
$$vO_2 = 0.003\, pO_2$$

References

1. West JB. Respiratory physiology. 9th ed. Philadelphia: Lippincott Williams and Wilkins; 2012.
2. Habibzadeh F, Yadollahie M. Temperature correction of the calculated alveolar oxygen tension. Anesthesiology. 1998;89(4):1042. https://doi.org/10.1097/00000542-199810000-00040.
3. Messina Z, Patrick H. Partial pressure of carbon dioxide. Treasure Island, FL: StatPearls; 2020.
4. Kaufman DP, Kandle PF, Murray I, Dhamoon AS. Physiology, oxyhemoglobin dissociation curve. Treasure Island, FL: StatPearls; 2020.

What Happens in a Person

4

4.1 Introduction

The daily rate of production of non-volatile (non-carbonic) acids is about 1 mEq/kg of body weight, which is closely related to dietary intake of protein, phospholipid, and endogenous protein catabolism. Non-volatile acids also arise from incomplete oxidation of carbohydrate and fat, which generates lactic acid and ketoacids. Despite this acid load, the arterial blood *pH* is sustained within the narrow range of 7.35–7.45. This could not be possible without close cooperation among the lungs, kidneys, and buffer systems.

4.2 Pulmonary Ventilation, Perfusion, and Blood-Gas Exchange

The primary function of the lungs is to preserve the oxygen and carbon dioxide content of the arterial blood within a relatively narrow range, which is essential for life. Lungs perform this function by allowing venous blood to come into contact with the alveolar air [1]. The contact surface (blood-gas interface) is tremendously large. There are three fundamental mechanisms involved in gas exchange:

1. Ventilation
2. Diffusion
3. Perfusion

4.2.1 Ventilation

The ventilatory function of the lungs depends on various factors, including lung volume, resistance of airways, elastic qualities (compliance) of the lungs and chest

F. Habibzadeh et al., *Pathophysiologic Basis of Acid-Base Disorders*,
https://doi.org/10.1007/978-981-16-0526-0_4

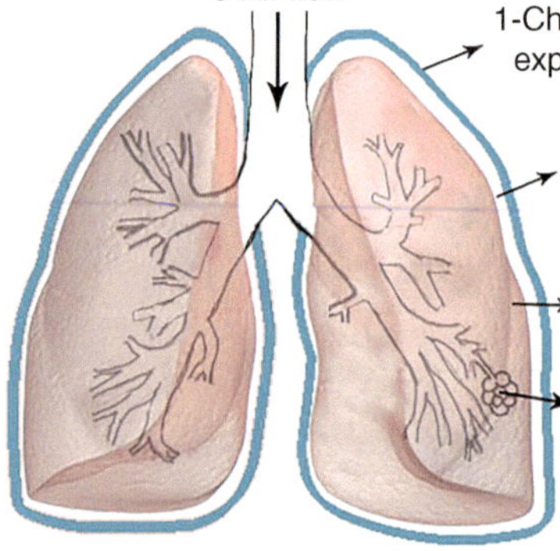

Fig. 4.1 The five sequential steps involving in a normal inspiration

wall, and pressure gradient between the mouth and the alveolar space. When there is no air flow, both mouth and alveolar pressures are equal to the atmospheric pressure.

During inspiration, the thoracic cage expands, the diaphragm descends and as a result, the pressure of the pleural space falls; this leads to inflation of the lungs, and in turn, causes an increase in alveolar volume and a decrease in alveolar pressure. As a consequence, the air flows into the alveoli (Fig. 4.1). Contrary to this, depending on elastic recoil of the lungs and chest wall, expiration is mainly passive.

As was remarked earlier, the pressure that acts upon the lungs and causes them to inflate during inspiration is the pleural cavity pressure. Normally, this pressure is negative relative to atmospheric pressure and, during normal breathing, changes between −5 (expiration) and −9 (inspiration) cm of water.

In an upright position, there is a pressure gradient in the pleural space from top to bottom. This pressure gradient is mainly gravity-dependent (i.e., in supine position, this gradient is from anterior to the posterior part of the lungs). This gradient is thought to be attributed to the weight of the lung. The pleural space pressure raises from the apex to the base (in an upright person). There is a pressure gradient of about 7–8 cm of water from the top to the bottom of the lung. This gradient largely affects the regional ventilation and perfusion, which will be discussed later in more detail.

4.2.1.1 Regional Distribution of Ventilation

The lung is hung within the chest wall. Therefore, the intrapleural pressure is not uniform—there is a vertical pressure gradient (in the upright person), with a progressive decline in pressure from the base (where the lung weight applies its effect entirely) to the apex of the lung (where the lung weight has no effect). As the pressure gradient between pleural cavity and atmosphere is more negative at the apex, the alveoli in the upper zone tend to be more expanded than those in the basilar part. It looks like a loosely coiled spring which, when suspended by its uppermost part, becomes gradually more expanded by its own weight from bottom to top (Fig. 4.2).

In the same way, in the supine position, the anterior alveoli are more inflated than those in the dependent posterior area. Therefore, in a supine person, the difference

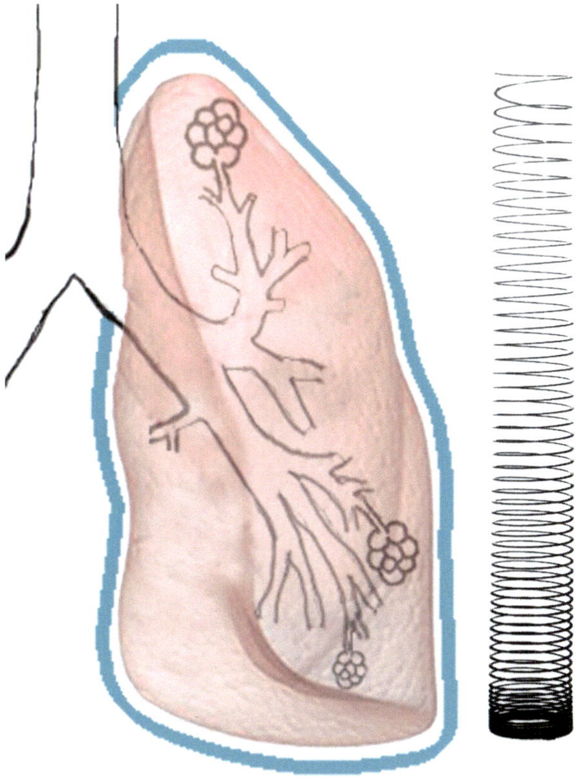

Fig. 4.2 Lung looks like a loosely coiled spring suspended by its uppermost coil

in alveolar expansion occurs antro-posteriorly. Due to these regional dissimilarities in alveolar expansion, the lung compliance of the more expanded upper zone is less than that of the lower zones in the upright posture. Therefore, basal ventilation exceeds that of apices [1].

Regional ventilation may be perturbed by small airway obstruction (e.g., by mucus plaque). This may result in a reduction in arterial partial pressure of oxygen.

4.2.2 Perfusion and Its Regional Distribution

Radioactive tracer techniques have revealed that pulmonary perfusion (blood flow) is not uniformly distributed, and like ventilation, it has a vertical gradient. Pulmonary perfusion per unit volume of lung tissue decreases from base to apex in the upright position. The lesser apical perfusion is due to the pressure drop caused by gravity. The blood pressure in the apical arterioles (which have higher height than the right ventricle [RV]) is just sufficient to open the capillary bed, only in systole. Therefore, there is a pulsatile flow (in systole) in the apices. In contrast, the blood pressure in the basilar arterioles (which have a lower height than RV) is higher than RV pressure, thus maintaining a continuous flow, which is about 10 times greater than that of the apical capillary bed (Fig. 4.3) [1].

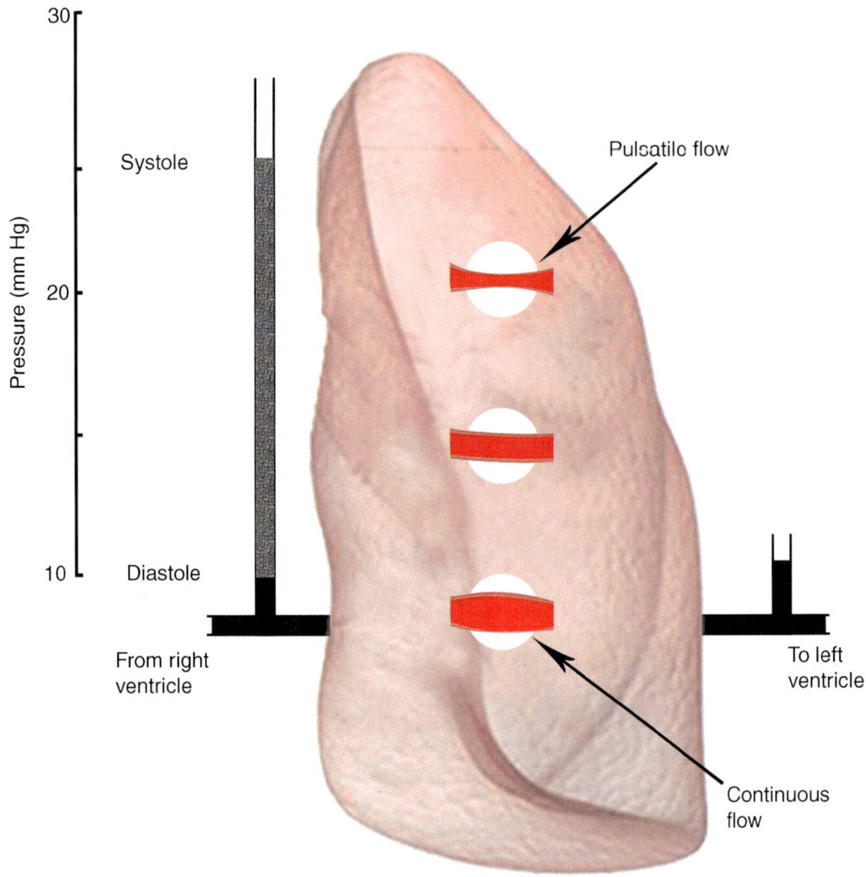

Fig. 4.3 Pulmonary capillary perfusion in various parts of the lung

In health, the oncotic pressure of the plasma protein (25 mm Hg) is higher than the mean intracapillary hydrostatic pressure, even at the bases of the lungs, which retains the fluid in vessels. Nevertheless, a moderate increase in pulmonary venous pressure (e.g., in left heart failure) elevates the intracapillary hydrostatic pressure enough to cause oozing of intravascular fluid into the interstitial fluid leading to pulmonary edema; this is obviously first seen at the bases.

4.2.3 Regional Variation in the Matching of Ventilation and Perfusion

As previously mentioned, in a normal lung, both alveolar ventilation ($\dot{V}$), and perfusion ($\dot{Q}$) change regionally in the same direction. If we divide the lung into a series of horizontal slices and compare apical and basilar slices, a two-fold increase

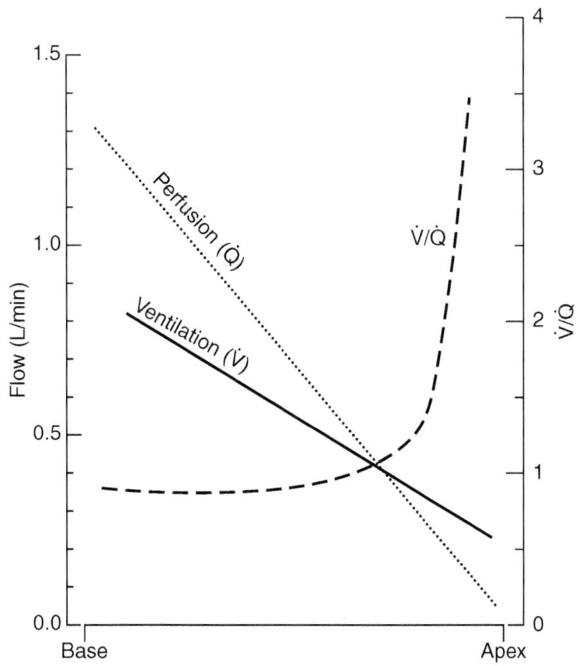

Fig. 4.4 Distribution of ventilation and perfusion in lung

in ventilation and ten-fold rise in perfusion per unit of lung volume will be detected. As a result, the regional matching of ventilation ($\dot{V}$) to perfusion ($\dot{Q}$), which may be represented as $\dot{V}/\dot{Q}$ ratio, is not uniform. The rate of increase of perfusion from apex to base is steeper than that for ventilation, thus, $\dot{V}/\dot{Q}$ decreases down the length of the lung from apex to base. The mean $\dot{V}/\dot{Q}$ ratio for a normal upright lung with a cardiac output of about 6 L/min, and alveolar ventilation of 5 L/min, lies between 0.8 and 0.9 [1]. However, regional $\dot{V}/\dot{Q}$ ratios vary significantly, from approximately 3.3 at the apex to 0.6 at the lung base (Fig. 4.4).

Apparently, apical alveoli are grossly overventilated, whereas basilar ones are relatively overperfused. The higher apical $\dot{V}/\dot{Q}$ ratio causes an alveolar oxygen tension, and hence tissue O_2 partial pressure, over 40 mm Hg higher than that at the lung base. Most gas exchange occurs in the lower part of the lungs, where $\dot{V}/\dot{Q}$ ratio deviates to a lesser extent from a perfect match than that in the upper zone. A disturbance in ventilation and perfusion match ($\dot{V}/\dot{Q}$ mismatch) is responsible for many major hypoxic states. The $\dot{V}/\dot{Q}$ mismatch, shunt, and related subjects will be discussed in more detail later.

4.3 Blood-Gas Interface and Gas Exchange

Figure 4.5 is a highly simplified diagram of the blood-gas interface. Oxygen and carbon dioxide, like other gases, move between alveolar air and blood by *simple diffusion*; they move from an area with higher partial pressure to an area with lower

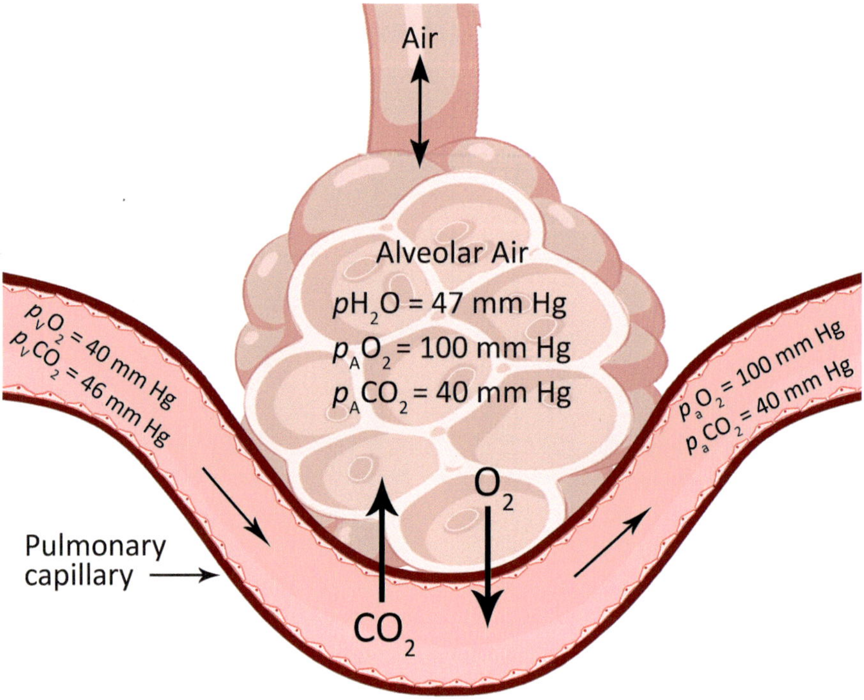

Fig. 4.5 Blood-gas interface in lung

partial pressure. Under normal circumstances, this system reaches an equilibrium state by the time the red cell (RBC) is only one-third of its way along the pulmonary capillary. The difference in pO_2 between alveolar gas and end-capillary blood is infinitesimally small—an insignificant fraction of 1 mm Hg.

The thickness of the blood-gas barrier is less than 0.5 μm. In certain disease states, the thickness of the blood-gas interface may be increased by edema, fluid, fibrous tissue, and the presence of inflammatory cells. This disturbs gas diffusion and may lead to *hypoxemia*. The *carbon dioxide penetration through the blood-gas interface is about 20 times more than that of oxygen*, and this is why diffuse pulmonary fibrotic or granulomatous diseases, such as asbestosis, which are associated with the impaired diffusion of oxygen, do not significantly affect the diffusion of CO_2 to cause an increase in arterial pCO_2. By the time this stage is reached, the arterial pO_2 is too depressed to be compatible with life. A raised alveolar pCO_2 usually means alveolar hypoventilation.

The surface area available for diffusion depends on the number of functioning alveoli. In an average male individual, it is about 70 m^2. The loss of diffusion surface area occurs in many pulmonary disorders. For example, in emphysema following the resection of alveoli, the diffusion surface area is diminished, and this causes hypoxemia.

4.4 Respiratory Quotient

The respiratory quotient (or respiratory exchange ratio), R, is defined as the ratio between the rate of CO_2 output and the rate of oxygen uptake, that is:

$$R = \frac{\text{Rate of } CO_2 \text{ output}}{\text{Rate of } O_2 \text{ uptake}}$$

The normal carriage of oxygen from the lung to the tissues by each deciliter (100 mL) of blood is approximately 5 mL, while the normal transport of carbon dioxide from the tissues to the lungs is about 4 mL per 100 mL of blood. Thus, under normal conditions, only about 80% as much carbon dioxide is expired from the lungs as there is oxygen uptake by the lungs. Using our definition for R, we have:

$$R = \frac{4 \text{ mL } CO_2 \text{ / dL of blood}}{5 \text{ mL } O_2 \text{ / dL of blood}} = 0.8$$

The value for R changes under various conditions. For example, if a person consumes foods composed only of carbohydrates, each oxygen molecule reacts with carbohydrates to form one molecule of CO_2, thus R rises to 1. Whereas, when one eats foods composed of only fats, some oxygen molecules form water instead of CO_2, thus R falls to about 0.7 [1]. For a person on a normal diet with an ordinary carbohydrate, fat, and protein content, the mean value for R is about 0.8.

4.5 Alveolar Air Composition

CO_2 can pass through the blood-gas barrier easily. Therefore, the partial pressure of CO_2 in the alveolar space (p_ACO_2) can be assumed to be just equal to the CO_2 tension in the arterial blood (p_aCO_2), which is normally around 40 mm Hg. This gives us a clue for calculating the alveolar partial pressure of oxygen (p_AO_2). A decline in alveolar pO_2 must be expected due to oxygen uptake. Using the definition for respiratory quotient (R), it can be stated that the alveolar pO_2 drops by the value p_ACO_2/R; that is, the alveolar pO_2 is

$$p_AO_2 = p_IO_2 - \frac{p_ACO_2}{R}$$

where p_IO_2 is the partial pressure of oxygen in the airways (where no gas exchange has yet occurred). In Fig. 4.6, the compositions of ambient and alveolar air are compared.

Example An arterial blood sample is analyzed for pCO_2 and pO_2. The resultant values are

$$p_aCO_2 = 40 \text{ mm Hg}$$
$$p_aO_2 = 70 \text{ mm Hg}$$

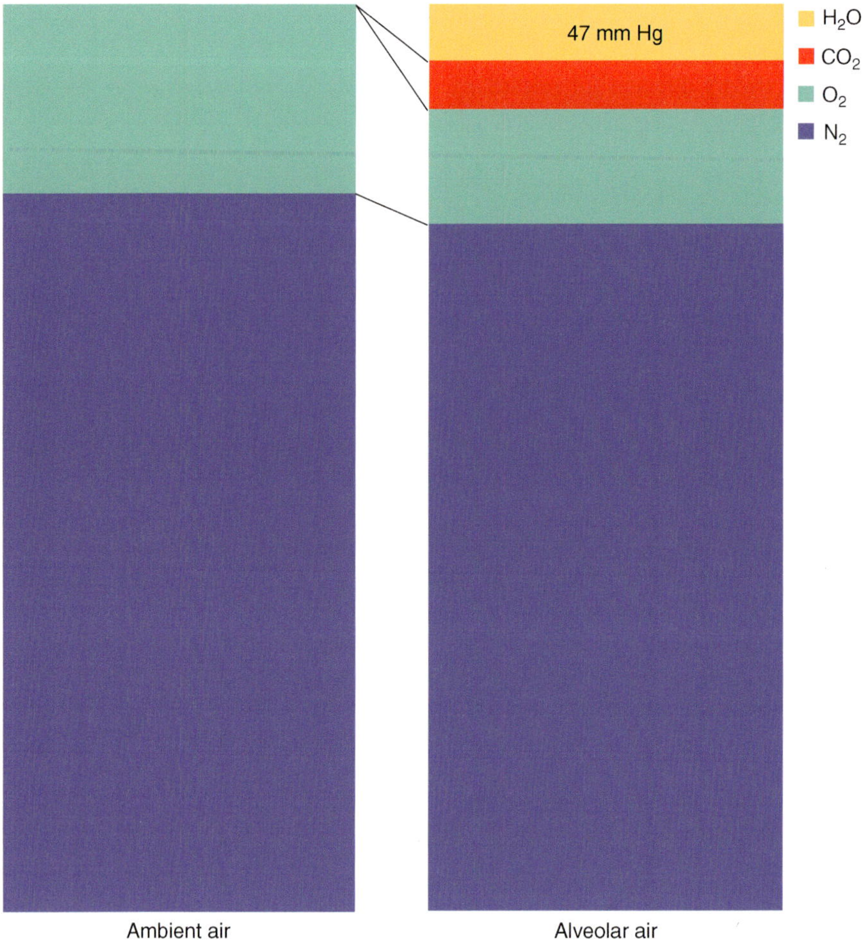

Fig. 4.6 Composition of the alveolar air compared with the ambient air. Note that while the partial pressure of carbon dioxide and water vapor is very low in the ambient air, they are important components of alveolar air

If the patient breaths ambient air, under a barometric pressure of 640 mm Hg, what is the p_AO_2 at the body temperature of 37 °C?

Solution: As CO_2 can pass through the blood-gas barrier easily, the p_ACO_2 is the same as p_aCO_2. For alveolar pO_2 then, we have

$$p_AO_2 = f_iO_2\left(p_B - p_{H_2O}\right) - \frac{p_aCO_2}{R}$$

Therefore:

$$p_{\mathrm{A}}\mathrm{O}_2 = \frac{21}{100}(640-47) - \frac{40}{0.8}$$
$$= 74.5\,\mathrm{mm\ Hg}$$

Obviously, there is a difference between alveolar and arterial oxygen tension, which in this case, is 4.5 (= 74.5–70) mm Hg. This *alveoli-arterial oxygen tension difference* is usually because of ventilation-perfusion mismatch and averages 8 mm Hg in normal young persons and increases in a linear fashion with age. It can reach up to 24 mm Hg in the 7th and 8th decades of life.

Example The $p_a CO_2$ and the body temperature of a person are assumed to be 40 mm Hg and 37 °C, respectively. Determine the barometric pressure under which the $p_A O_2$ falls to zero!

Solution:

$$p_{\mathrm{A}}\mathrm{O}_2 = f_i\mathrm{O}_2\left(p_{\mathrm{B}} - p_{\mathrm{H_2O}}\right) - \frac{p_{\mathrm{a}}\mathrm{CO}_2}{R}$$
$$0 = 0.21(p_{\mathrm{B}} - 47) - \frac{40}{0.8}$$
$$0 = 0.21\,p_{\mathrm{B}} - 9.87 - 50$$

Therefore:

$$p_{\mathrm{B}} = 285\,\mathrm{mm\ Hg}$$

At the altitude of 15000 m, the atmospheric pressure is about 285 mm Hg, and accordingly, the alveolar oxygen tension is zero! Actually this is not the case, and *body responds to hypoxemia by hyperventilation and lowering the alveolar pCO_2.*

Example If the person in the previous example (at 15000 m) breaths 70% oxygen, then calculate the $p_A O_2$.

Solution:

$$p_{\mathrm{A}}\mathrm{O}_2 = \frac{70}{100}(285-47) - \frac{40}{0.8}$$
$$= 116.6\,\mathrm{mm\ Hg}$$

Example When a diver descends, the pressure of the surrounding water, and therefore of the gas he breaths, is augmented by about 760 mm Hg for each 10 m of depth. What is the $p_A O_2$ of a person who is at 90-m depth and breaths 21% oxygen? Suppose the $p_a CO_2$ and body temperature to be 40 mm Hg and 37 °C, respectively.

Solution: Under the water, the pressure of the breathing gas has two components, a part of which owing to atmospheric pressure over the water (760 mm Hg), the other due to the water weight, that is:

$$p_{\mathrm{Water}} = \frac{\mathrm{Depth}_{(\mathrm{m})}}{10} \times 760\,\mathrm{mm\ Hg}$$

Therefore:

$$\begin{aligned} p_{\text{amb}} &= p_{\text{atmospheric}} + p_{\text{Water}} \\ &= 760 + \left(\frac{90}{10} \times 760 \right) \\ &= 760 + 6840 \\ &= 7600\,\text{mm Hg} \end{aligned}$$

and

$$\begin{aligned} p_{\text{A}}\text{O}_2 &= f_i\text{O}_2 \left(p_{\text{amb}} - p_{\text{H}_2\text{O}} \right) - \frac{p_{\text{a}}\text{CO}_2}{R} \\ &= 0.21\left(7600 - 47\right) - \frac{40}{0.8} \\ &\approx 1536\,\text{mm Hg} \end{aligned}$$

This is definitely unnecessarily high for hemoglobin saturation and is, *in any case, toxic*.

Example Find out the fraction of oxygen in the breathing gas ($f_i O_2$) which preserves an alveolar pO_2 of 100 mm Hg in the case of the diver in the previous example.

Solution: Considering the previous example, we have:

$$p_{\text{A}}\text{O}_2 = f_i\text{O}_2 \left(7600 - 47\right) - \frac{40}{0.8}$$

Therefore:

$$100 = 7553 \times f_i O_2 - 50$$

Consequently:

$$f_i\text{O}_2 = 0.02 \;\left(\text{Only } 2\%!\right)$$

4.6 Carriage of O_2 by the Blood

The most important purpose of the cardiopulmonary system is the transport of oxygen to the tissues and removal of the carbon dioxide resulting from the metabolism. A pO_2 of about 2 mm Hg should be sustained within the cells to maintain their oxidative metabolism. Based on Henry's law, the amount of dissolved oxygen is proportional to the partial pressure of oxygen. The solubility coefficient of oxygen in blood, as remarked in the previous chapter, is 0.003 mL/dL per mm Hg.

Example What is the volume of the dissolved oxygen in 100 mL of blood, if the partial pressure of oxygen in the alveoli is 100 mm Hg?

Solution: For simplicity, the partial pressure of oxygen in the pulmonary end-capillary blood can be taken to be the same as that in the alveolar space. Thus, the dissolved oxygen can be determined simply as:

$$\begin{aligned} vO_2 &= s\ p_aO_2 \\ &= 0.003 \times 100 \\ &= 0.3\,\text{mL } O_2/\text{dL of blood} \end{aligned}$$

The oxygen needs of a normal resting subject is about 300 mL/min. If the tissues can uptake all the dissolved oxygen from the blood, and if one depends only on dissolved oxygen, the amount of cardiac output must then be about 100 L/min, a level unacceptable to maintain. This obstacle is overcome by the *reversible binding of oxygen to hemoglobin.*

Hemoglobin is a tetramer (two α and two β chains in adult) composed of a globulin molecule and four heme molecules, each of which can react reversibly with a single oxygen molecule to form oxyhemoglobin according to the reversible reaction:

$$Hb + O_2 \rightleftharpoons HbO_2 \tag{4.1}$$

It should be remarked that *oxygenation of hemoglobin is not an oxidation reaction*, and the iron atom in both hemoglobin and oxyhemoglobin is in the reduced or ferrous state. Hemoglobin whose iron is oxidized to the ferric state is unable to transport oxygen and is called *methemoglobin*. Some substances, including some nitrates, can transform hemoglobin to methemoglobin, and this is why these materials can result in severe hypoxic states.

The binding capacity of hemoglobin is about 1.34 mL of oxygen per gram of hemoglobin, but not all of the hemoglobin molecules carry oxygen. By definition, the percentage saturation of hemoglobin ($Hb_{\text{Sat\%}}$) is:

$$Hb_{\text{Sat\%}} = \frac{HbO_2}{HbO_2 + Hb} \times 100$$

The correlation between percentage saturation and the partial pressure of oxygen is represented as the *dissociation curve of hemoglobin*, which is discovered experimentally. In general, *blood oxygen content* can be determined by the following formula:

$$\begin{aligned} O_2\ \text{Content} &= Hb\text{-bounded}\ O_2 + \text{Disolved}\ O_2 \\ &= 1.34\left[Hb\right]\frac{Hb_{\text{Sat\%}}}{100} + 0.003\ p_aO_2 \end{aligned}$$

where $[Hb]$ designates hemoglobin concentration in g/dL.

Example The hemoglobin concentration of whole blood is approximately 15 g/dL. Calculate the O_2 content of the blood, if the partial pressure of oxygen is 100 mm Hg.

Solution: $$O_2\ \text{Content} = 1.34\left[Hb\right]\frac{Hb_{\text{Sat\%}}}{100} + 0.003\ p_{\text{a}}O_2$$

The corresponding percentage saturation for a pO_2 of 100 mm Hg is 97.4, therefore:

$$\begin{aligned} O_2\ \text{Content} &= 1.34 \times 15 \times \frac{97.4}{100} + 0.003 \times 100 \\ &= 19.9\,\text{mL/dL of blood} \end{aligned}$$

Now, assuming the O_2 content of 19.9 mL/dL of blood, and a normal resting oxygen requirement of about 300 mL/min, the required cardiac output can be easily calculated to be about 1.5 L/min.

4.6.1 Oxyhemoglobin Dissociation Curve

The oxygenation of each heme molecule in the tetramer alters the oxygen affinity of the other subunits and is usually referred to as a *heme-heme interaction* [2, 3]. The heme-heme interaction is responsible for the sigmoid shape of the oxyhemoglobin dissociation curve (Fig. 4.7). The p_{50} is defined as the partial pressure of oxygen (pO_2) at which hemoglobin is 50% saturated.

The sigmoid shape of the oxyhemoglobin dissociation curve provides significant physiological consequences. The upper portion of the curve is relatively flat. A fall in oxygen tension in this zone (e.g., from 100 to 60 mm Hg) will produce a relatively small fall in hemoglobin oxygen saturation, thus a modest decline in O_2 content. Consequently, persons who live at high altitudes (e.g., 3000 m), where the alveolar pO_2 is low (e.g., 60 mm Hg at an altitude of about 3000 m), still sustain oxygen saturation of about 90%, which is clearly enough to overcome their oxygen requirements. Conversely, an increase in pO_2 of arterial blood in this range causes only a slight rise in oxygen saturation. As a result, breathing of the air with high O_2 percentage (f_iO_2) causes the breather to be incapable of compensating hypoxemia resulting from areas of impaired gas exchange in the lung.

The lower, steeper zone of the hemoglobin dissociation curve also has physiological implications. In this part, a small decline in pO_2 of blood results in a relatively great drop in hemoglobin oxygen saturation, and consequently in blood oxygen content. Therefore, the transfer of oxygen from blood to metabolically active tissues is facilitated.

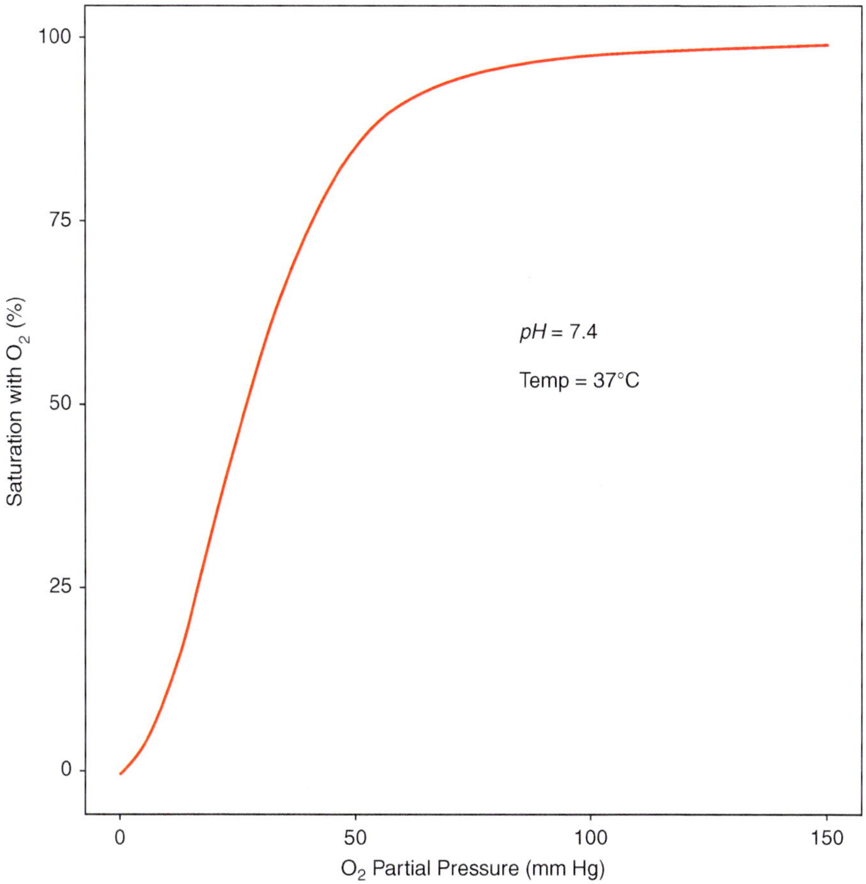

Fig. 4.7 Oxyhemoglobin dissociation curve

Example A 16-year-old boy presented with the chief complaint of easy fatigability. Laboratory examination revealed a blood hemoglobin concentration ($[Hb]$) of 7 g/dL and an arterial pO_2 of 100 mm Hg. Determine the amount of oxygen accessible to the tissues.

Solution:

$$O_2\ \text{Content} = 1.34[Hb]\frac{Hb_{\text{Sat\%}}}{100} + 0.003\ p_aO_2$$

The percentage saturation corresponding to p_aO_2 of 100 mm Hg is 97.4 (Fig. 4.7), therefore:

$$\begin{aligned} O_2\ \text{Content} &= 1.34 \times 7 \times \frac{97.4}{100} + 0.003 \times 100 \\ &= 9.4\ \text{mL/dL of blood} \end{aligned}$$

Example What will be the blood O_2 content in the patient in the previous example, if:

(a) the p_aO_2 is increased to 150 mm Hg (by raising f_iO_2)?
(b) the hemoglobin concentration is raised to 10 g/dL (by blood transfusion)?

Solution: (a) The percentage saturation corresponding to p_aO_2 of 150 mm Hg is 100 (Fig. 4.7), then:

$$\begin{aligned} O_2 \text{ Content} &= 1.34 \times 7 \times \frac{100}{100} + 0.003 \times 100 \\ &= 9.8 \text{ mL/dL of blood} \end{aligned}$$

(b) The percentage saturation corresponding to p_aO_2 of 100 mm Hg is 97.4 (Fig. 4.7), then:

$$\begin{aligned} O_2 \text{ Content} &= 1.34 \times 10 \times \frac{97.4}{100} + 0.003 \times 100 \\ &= 13.4 \text{ mL/dL of blood} \end{aligned}$$

Consequently, *in a patient with anemia, the best way for augmentation of tissue oxygenation is to increase the hemoglobin concentration* (i.e., *blood transfusion*) *rather than raising the inspired oxygen concentration.*

4.6.1.1 Factors Affecting the Oxyhemoglobin Dissociation Curve

Several factors can alter the relation between pO2 and hemoglobin saturation. These factors can shift the oxyhemoglobin dissociation saturation curve to either the right or the left, so that the upper flat zone of the curve, corresponding to high hemoglobin saturation, is either condensed or expanded, respectively (Fig. 4.8).

These shifts can be described in terms of p_{50}; a right shift resulting in a rise in p_{50}, whereas a left shift causes it to fall. The most significant of these factors are *pH*; pCO_2; 2,3-diphosphoglycerate (2,3-DPG) concentration; and temperature.

Although, at first glance, it seems that an increased p_{50} due to a right shift (Fig. 4.8, curve 3) is unfavorable, since a smaller amount of oxygen is being transferred for a given pO_2, a careful look at the diagram discloses that, as a result of the shape of curve 3 (condensed upper flat zone), an elevated p_{50} indicates that, for a given decline in arterial pO_2 in the physiologic range, a greater amount of oxygen becomes accessible to the tissues.

The pO_2 of the arterial blood, which is about 90 mm Hg, drops to 40 mm Hg, after passing through the systemic capillaries. According to curve 2 (Fig. 4.8, the solid green curve), this decline in pO_2 causes the oxygen saturation to decrease only by 20%, whereas if curve 3 (dashed red curve) is employed, the fall in oxygen saturation is 40%.

When hemoglobin is oxygenated, hydrogen ions are liberated from the molecule. The increase in hydrogen ion concentration (i.e., reduction in *pH*) is an external stress for this system. Considering Le Chatelier's principle, the system responds in

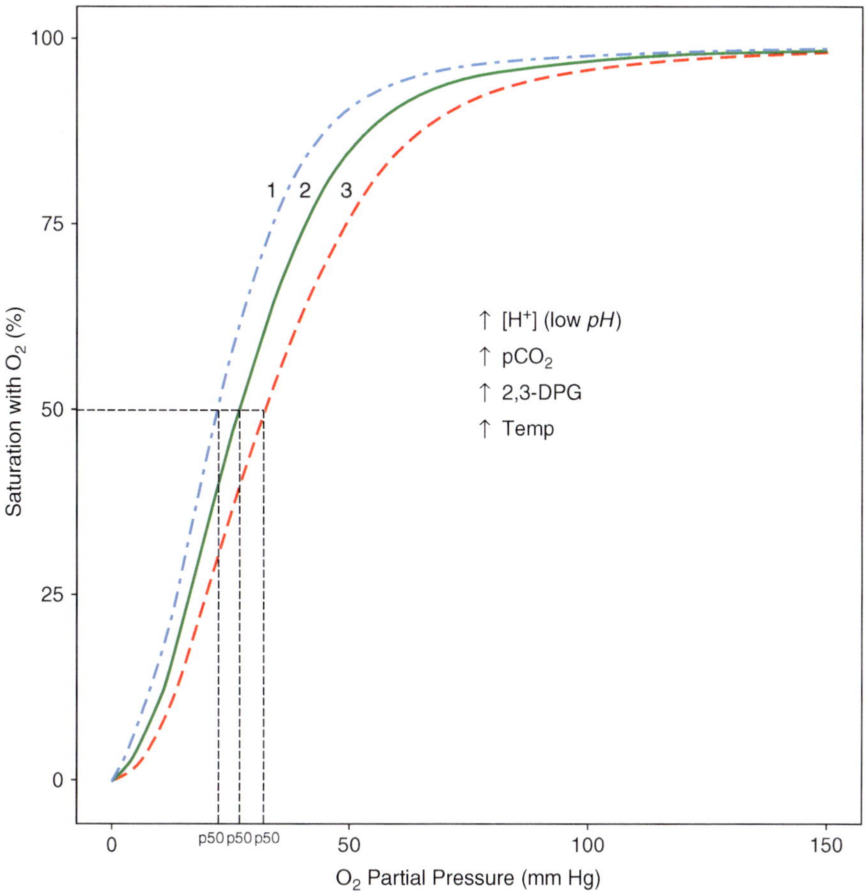

Fig. 4.8 Factors that can shift the oxyhemoglobin dissociation curve

such a way as to minimize the influence of external stress. Therefore, after a decrease in *pH*, the process of oxygenation of hemoglobin tends to reverse and the hemoglobin returns to its deoxygenated state with the release of oxygen. Metabolically active tissues, such as exercising muscles, make up a more acidic environment for the blood as a consequent of the local production of CO_2 and lactic acid; this low *pH* enhances the transfer of oxygen to the tissues for the same fall in pO_2. In other words, a decrease in *pH* causes an increase in p_{50}, or shift of oxyhemoglobin dissociation curve to the right, a phenomenon which is called the *Bohr effect* [4].

The partial pressure of CO_2 also influences the hemoglobin dissociation curve. It can be shown that a rise in pCO_2, per se, can shift the hemoglobin dissociation curve to the right, an effect independent of *pH*. Organic phosphates combine with basic groups of hemoglobin. The organic phosphate 2,3-diphosphoglycerate (2,3-DPG) is an intermediate in erythrocyte carbohydrate metabolism and composes most of the phosphate in red cells. The concentration of 2,3-DPG in human erythrocytes is around 0.8 mol/mol of hemoglobin. If the concentration of 2,3-DPG is increased, it competes with oxygen for binding sites on deoxygenated hemoglobin, thereby, reducing its oxygen affinity, causing the hemoglobin dissociation curve to shift to the right. The level of 2,3-DPG is adjusted by enzymatic reactions which are *pH*-dependent, so that acidity or alkalinity tends to suppress or stimulate its production, respectively. An acute decline in plasma *pH* results in a sudden shift of the oxyhemoglobin dissociation curve to the right. If this fall persists for several hours, the low plasma *pH* suppresses the 2,3-DPG generation. The low 2,3-DPG level applies a counterbalancing effect on the *pH*-mediated right shift of the curve. Therefore, when chronic long-standing acidosis is rapidly corrected with bicarbonate, the influence of *pH* on the curve (right shift) disappears, while the remaining low 2,3-DPG level may have a noxious *overshoot effect* by raising the oxygen affinity of hemoglobin, and reducing its supply to the tissues.

Temperature also alters the hemoglobin dissociation curve, so that an increase in temperature of blood shifts the curve to the right, and therefore, decreases the hemoglobin oxygen affinity. This enhances the oxygenation of the metabolized tissues, the temperature of which is a little higher than that of the lungs. Cold skin may be bright pink, not only because cold diminishes the rate of oxygen consumption, but also because hemoglobin binds oxygen more firmly in the cold.

Deoxygenated hemoglobin is a weaker acid, and therefore, relatively alkaline. Consequently, the presence of deoxygenated hemoglobin stimulates the generation of 2,3-DPG with the sequential shift of the curve to the right. This circumstance is usually associated with long-standing hypoxemic states such as cyanotic heart disease or chronic bronchitis. In other conditions, 2,3-DPG may be depleted with a consequent left shift of the curve and decline in blood oxygen transferring capacity. These conditions include storage of blood for transfusion, hypophosphatemia, and the elevated blood level of carboxyhemoglobin associated with cigarette smoking.

4.7 Carriage of Carbon Dioxide

Carbon dioxide diffuses under its partial pressure gradient from metabolizing tissues into the blood of capillaries perfusing them. Carbon dioxide is carried by the blood in three forms:

1. as dissolved CO_2 in plasma
2. as combined with hemoglobin
3. as bicarbonate

Plasma alone is an ineffective carrier of CO_2; only 5% of total carbon dioxide is carried in this way. The amount of dissolved CO_2, as discussed earlier, follows the well-known Henry's law. A small fraction of dissolved CO_2 in plasma reacts with water to produce carbonic acid (H_2CO_3), which is a weak acid. Carbonic acid then ionizes according to the equation:

$$H_2O + CO_2 \rightleftharpoons H_2CO_3 \rightleftharpoons H^+ + HCO_3^-$$

to form hydrogen ion (H^+) and bicarbonate (HCO_3^-). The above equation can be written as:

$$H_2O + CO_2 \rightleftharpoons H^+ + HCO_3^- \tag{4.2}$$

CO_2 is fat-soluble and diffuses into red blood cells (RBC), where the above reaction progresses rapidly as a result of the presence of *carbonic anhydrase*, an enzyme which catalyzes the above reactions. This causes a concentration gradient of bicarbonate between the red cell and the plasma, so that bicarbonate diffuses from the erythrocyte into the plasma. However, bicarbonate (HCO_3^-) is a negatively charged ion and its diffusion into the plasma perturbs the electrical neutrality of the erythrocyte and the plasma. To maintain the electrical neutrality of both the plasma and the red cell, either an equal number of positively charged cations should diffuse out of the red cell, or an equal number of negatively charged anions must diffuse from the plasma into the erythrocyte. During the very short period in which these reactions occur, the red cell membrane is relatively impermeable to cations; thus, inward diffusion of anions takes place. The anions available in plasma are chloride ions; chloride ions diffuse into the erythrocyte as bicarbonate ions diffuse out—a phenomenon known as the *chloride shift*. This exchange continues until equilibrium is achieved. Ninety percent of total blood carbon dioxide is carried as bicarbonate in this way. The remaining 5% combines reversibly with amino groups (–NH_2) on deoxygenated hemoglobin to form hemoglobin carbamate:

$$Hb\text{-}NH_2 + CO_2 \rightleftharpoons Hb\text{-}NHCOOH \rightleftharpoons H^+ + Hb\text{-}NHCOO^-$$

Then, the produced hydrogen ions (H^+) are buffered by hemoglobin. Figure 4.9 is a simplified illustration of the mode of carriage of carbon dioxide in the blood.

When venous blood in the lungs comes into contact with alveolar air, carbon dioxide in the plasma under its partial pressure gradient diffuses into the alveolar space. Recalling Le Chatelier's principle, it is obvious that all the chemical reactions in Fig. 4.9 proceed in the opposite direction, that is from right to left. Thus, *red blood cells are necessary not only for oxygen carriage, but also for* CO_2 *transport.*

4.8 Control of Respiration

Although the regulation of ventilation is very complex, a basic understanding of its physiologic function is essential for the interpretation of acid-base status. The neural centers controlling the respiration are chiefly located in the reticular formation of medulla oblongata, which are known as the medullary respiratory systems [1]. The output of these centers is in turn modulated by cortical and pontine activity, and by signals from peripheral chemoreceptors which are located in the aortic arch and

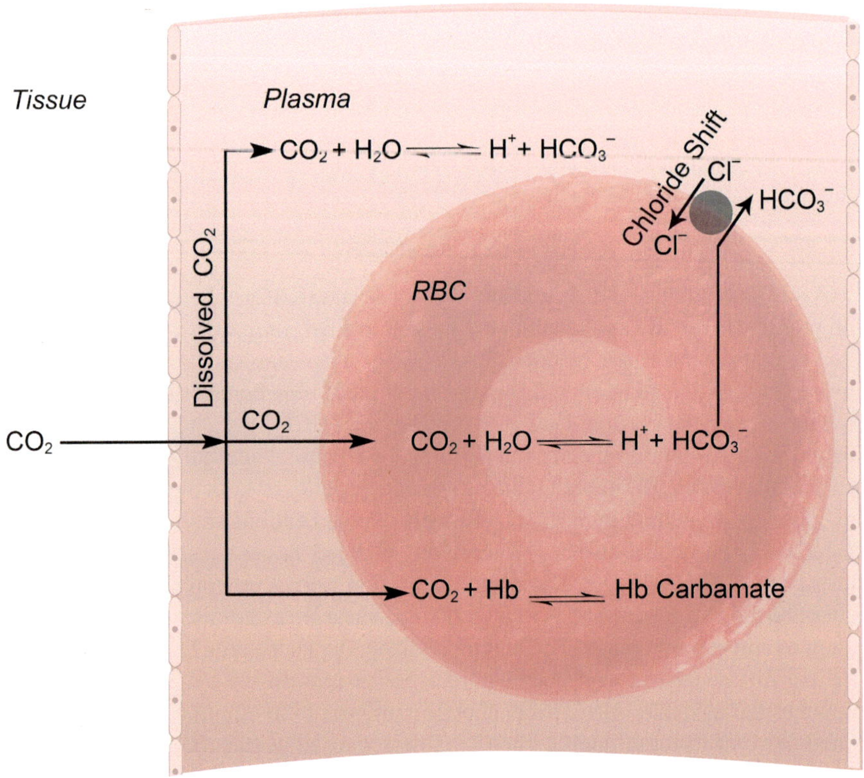

Fig. 4.9 Carriage of carbon dioxide in the blood

the carotid body. This *regulatory system is extremely sensitive to arterial* pCO_2 level, and a 5% rise in p_aCO_2 causes the minute ventilation to double. Carbon dioxide can cross the blood-brain barrier (BBB) more easily than can bicarbonate; then, CO_2 reacts with water to form carbonic acid, the consequent ionization of which to bicarbonate and hydrogen ions causes cerebrospinal fluid (CSF) to be more acidic (lowers *pH* of CSF). The medulla has receptors sensitive to H^+ on its ventral surface which when bathed with acid CSF (H^+) responds initially by raising the tidal volume and later by an increase in the respiratory rate. Prolonged acidity of the CSF, which may occur in *chronic obstructive pulmonary disease* (COPD), results in an augmented CSF bicarbonate concentration, which increases the *pH* of CSF again (look at the Henderson-Hasselbalch equation). Consequently, *a patient with an elevated arterial* pCO_2*, for example, due to chronic bronchitis, may have a reduced hyperventilatory response to carbon dioxide, and depends instead on* p_aO_2 *and hypoxic drive*. Uncontrolled oxygen therapy in such a patient may induce apnea by raising arterial pO_2 above the normal level of the patient, thereby leading to secondary hypoventilation and a further increase in p_aCO_2, which raises the intracranial pressure and acts as a respiratory depressant (CO_2 *narcosis*) [5].

The carotid body and aortic arch chemoreceptors are stimulated dominantly by hypoxia and, to a lesser extent, by hypercapnia. The carotid body chemoreceptors are also sensitive to a decline in *pH* (acidemia). These peripheral chemoreceptors are highly active metabolically, and it has been proposed that they are stimulated by the local accumulation of products of anaerobic metabolism, occurring either as a result of a decrease in arterial pO_2 (not O_2 content), or from diminished perfusion in the presence of normoxemia as may occur in hemorrhagic shock. Their afferent signals are carried to the medulla by the *glossopharyngeal* (IX) and *vagus* (X) nerves. The peripheral chemoreceptor response to hypoxia is not as sensitive as the medullary carbon dioxide response, and the alveolar pO_2 is usually diminished to about 50 mm Hg before the chemoreceptors take over. There are a few sensory nerve endings in the alveolar walls in juxtaposition to the pulmonary capillaries, hence, the name *J* receptors. Injection of irritant chemicals into the pulmonary blood stimulates these receptors. They can also be excited in conditions such as pulmonary edema, which may occur as a consequence of congestive heart failure (CHF).

An abnormal respiration called *Cheyne-Stokes* breathing is characterized by slowly waxing and waning respiration, repeating every 45 s to 3 min. The fundamental mechanism of Cheyne-Stokes breathing provides a clue to the function of the respiratory center [6].

Consider that respiration becomes much more rapid (tachypnea) and deeper (hyperventilation) than usual. This causes a rise in alveolar ventilation and, consequently, a fall in alveolar and pulmonary blood pCO_2. After a brief time, the pulmonary blood passes through the left ventricle and reaches the brain, and diminished p_aCO_2 begins to suppress the respiratory center. As a result, the pulmonary blood pCO_2 rises. After a further period of time, the blood carrying the elevated CO_2 arrives at the respiratory center and stimulates the respiration again, thus making the person overbreathe once again, and starting a new cycle of depressed respiration. The cycles thus continue on and on, causing Cheyne-Stokes periodic respiration.

The Cheyne-Stokes breathing is frequently seen in severe cardiac failure (CHF) associated with hypotension and following cerebrovascular accidents (CVA) [7]. This instability of the respiratory center may result from several factors, such as prolonged circulation time resulting in delayed feedback signals to the respiratory center, or from increased sensitivity of the CO_2 control system, as a result of damage to higher centers.

4.9 Buffers

From the previous chapter, it was learned that a buffer is a solution composed of an acid-base conjugate pair, and it functions at maximal capacity when the *pH* of the solution is around the *pK* of the buffer system.

The first line of defense in living organisms against alterations in their internal *pH* is provided by buffer systems. There are various buffer systems in the human body which preserve the internal *pH* within a confined range. These buffer systems are all in equilibrium with each other. Therefore, *a change in one buffer pair provokes changes in other buffer systems*. In other words, the hydrogen ion concentration can be corrected by manipulating the concentration of the components of a single buffer system.

One of the most important buffer systems is the carbonic acid-bicarbonate system. This system consists of carbonic acid (H_2CO_3), as the proton donor (conjugate acid), and bicarbonate (HCO_3^-), as the proton acceptor (conjugate base):

$$H_2CO_3 \rightleftharpoons H^+ + HCO_3^- \tag{4.3}$$

This system functions as a buffer similar to other conjugate acid-base pairs. However, what makes it unique is that one of its components, carbonic acid (H_2CO_3), can be generated from dissolved carbon dioxide and water, according to the reaction:

$$H_2O + CO_2 \rightleftharpoons H_2CO_3 \tag{4.4}$$

Considering Eqs. (4.3) and (4.4), we have:

$$H_2O + CO_2 \rightleftharpoons H^+ + HCO_3^- \tag{4.2}$$

The *pK* of the previous reaction at 37 °C is 6.1. According to the Henderson-Hasselbalch equation (Eq. (3.5)), with an α of 0.0301, then:

$$pH = 6.1 + \log \frac{\left[HCO_3^-\right]}{0.0301\, pCO_2}$$

The *pH* of a bicarbonate buffer system depends on the concentration of HCO_3^- and partial pressure of CO_2. Although the *pK* of this system is 6.1, *the bicarbonate system is the predominant buffer system in plasma and extracellular fluids,* and it is a potent physiological buffer near the normal plasma *pH* of 7.4 as the dissolved plasma CO_2 is in equilibrium with a large reserve capacity of gaseous CO_2 in the alveolar air, and the plasma bicarbonate concentration, which is regulated by the kidneys. When the *pH* of the blood declines (excess H^+), for example, in renal failure, some of the bicarbonate (HCO_3^-) reacts with excess H^+ to produce carbonic acid (H_2CO_3) (Eq. (4.3)). The resultant H_2CO_3 then dissociates to water and dissolved CO_2 (Eq. (4.4)), which in turn is delivered as the gaseous CO_2 into the alveolar air. Raised p_aCO_2 stimulates the respiratory center and causes hyperventilation and tachypnea (*respiratory response for acidosis*) which results in the removal of the excess CO_2 from the alveolar air.

In contrast, whenever the blood must absorb OH^- (high *pH*), for example, following ingestion of sodium bicarbonate, the surplus OH^- perturbs the chemical equilibrium of water and reacts with H^+ to form H_2O. The reduced hydrogen ion concentration in turn disturbs the equilibrium of the Eq. (4.3), thus, provoking the carbonic acid (H_2CO_3) decomposition to form bicarbonate (HCO_3^-) and H^+. The decreased carbonic acid concentration causes the Eq. (4.4) to proceed to the right side to form carbonic acid, at the expense of the dissolved CO_2. The low pCO_2, in conjunction with the high *pH*, inhibits the respiratory center, producing hypoventilation and bradypnea (*respiratory response for alkalosis*) which result in CO_2

retention. As blood passes through the many fine capillaries in the lungs, its bicarbonate buffer system promptly comes into near equilibrium with the CO_2 in the alveolar air. The cooperation between the bicarbonate buffer system and the action of the lungs provides a highly efficient mechanism for sustaining the blood *pH* at a notably constant normal value of 7.4.

Another significant buffer is the phosphate buffer system. This system is composed of dihydrogen phosphate ion ($H_2PO_4^-$) as the proton donor (conjugate acid), and monohydrogen phosphate ion (HPO_4^{2-}) as the proton acceptor (conjugate base):

$$H_2PO_4^- \rightleftharpoons H^+ + HPO_4^{2-} \quad (4.5)$$

The *pK* of this reaction at 37 °C is 6.86. The phosphate buffer pair $H_2PO_4^-$ and HPO_4^{2-} tends to oppose alterations in *pH* in the range of about 6.1–7.7 and is therefore competent in providing buffering ability in intracellular fluid, whose normal *pH* is in the range 6.9–7.4.

The ammonia-ammonium conjugate pair is also a buffer system:

$$NH_4^+ \rightleftharpoons H^+ + NH_3 \quad (4.6)$$

The *pK* of this reaction is approximately 9.25. *The ammonia and phosphate are typically the only important urinary buffers* and will be discussed in more detail later.

Two other compounds with buffering capacity are those substances with carboxyl group (–COOH) and amino group (–NH_2). They react according to the reversible reactions:

$$\text{R-COOH} \rightleftharpoons H^+ + \text{R-COO}^-$$

and

$$\text{R-NH}_3^+ \rightleftharpoons H^+ + \text{R-NH}_2$$

where the letter R depicts any other group which may be attached to the carbon atom.

Imidazole group can also possess buffering action according to the reaction:

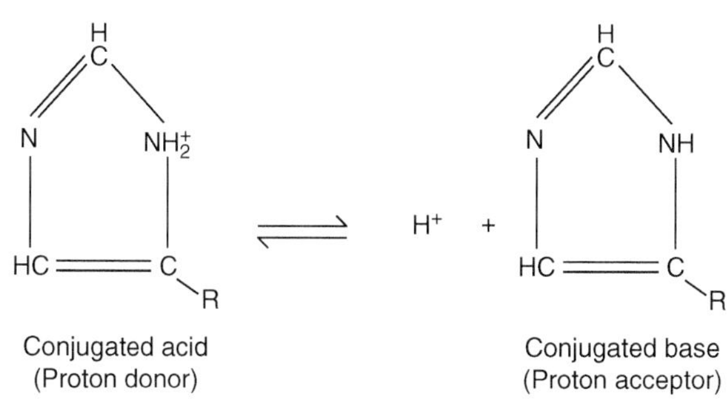

Amino acids are buffers because all are composed of carboxyl and amino groups; some (e.g., histidine) contain the imidazole group. A protein such as hemoglobin, which is made up of amino acids, has a buffering activity because its molecule

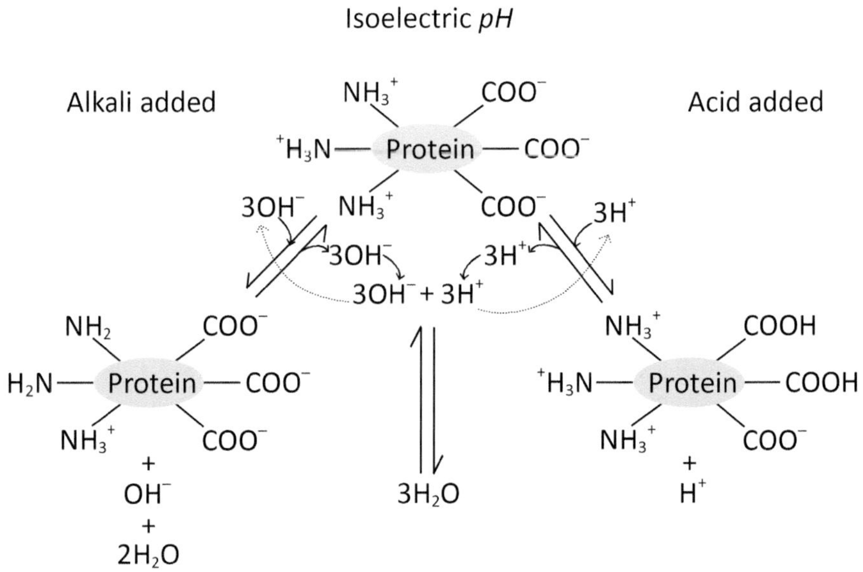

Fig. 4.10 Buffering action of proteins

contains a large number of acidic and basic groups—carboxyl (–COOH), amino (–NH_2), and guanido (–NH–CNH–NH_2) groups. The imidazole group of histidine also contributes to the buffering ability of the proteins (Fig. 4.10).

At the isoelectric *pH*, the isoionic protein is demonstrated as having three acidic and three basic groups (Fig. 4.10). When three hydrogen ions are added to the solution, two of the hydrogen ions combine with the basic carboxyl groups (–COO^-), developing undissociated groups (–COOH). One of the hydrogen ions remains in solution, making it more acidic. Had the protein not existed, all three hydrogen ions would have persisted in the solution, and the solution's acidity would have been greater. On the other hand, when hydroxyl ions are added to the solution, some of the acidic groups donate their hydrogen ions, which combine with the hydroxyl groups to make water. The increase in alkalinity of the solution is not as prominent as it would have been had the protein not been present. In this way, protein buffers the solution, opposing changes in hydrogen ion concentration when acid is added to or eliminated from the solution. Much of the buffering power of oxyhemoglobin in the physiologic range is done by imidazole groups, especially the C-terminal ones of the β chains. Also, the α amino groups of the α chains, which are not combined with CO_2 or with 2,3-DPG, participate in the buffering ability in the physiologic range. As the oxyhemoglobin releases its oxygen at the tissue, it becomes a weaker acid ($pK = 7.71$) which permits it to accept H^+, a phenomenon known as the *Haldane effect*. In contrary, the oxygenation of hemoglobin causes it to become a stronger acid ($pK = 6.17$), and therefore, leads to the release of H^+ into the blood. Over the physiologic range of *pH*, for one *pH* unit change, for every milliequivalent of hemoglobin (16.7 g), 7.2 millimoles of acid should be added to or removed from the solution.

Example 1000 mL of human oxyhemoglobin solution with a pCO_2 of 40 mm Hg, and an oxyhemoglobin concentration of 14 g/dL is kept at 37 °C. If the *pH* of the solution is 7.26, what is the final *pH*, after the addition of 10 mmol of hydrochloric acid?

Solution: 16.7 g of hemoglobin is one milliequivalent (mEq); therefore, the hemoglobin concentration of our solution is:

$$\frac{14}{16.7} = 0.838\,\text{mEq} / \text{dL}$$
$$= 8.38\,\text{mEq} / \text{L}$$

The addition of 7.2 mmol of acid to a similar solution with a hemoglobin concentration of 1 mEq/L causes the *pH* to fall by 1 unit, thus the addition of 10 mmol of acid to a solution with hemoglobin concentration of 8.38 mEq/L will cause the *pH* to decrease by:

$$\frac{\left(\frac{10}{7.2}\right)}{8.38} = 0.17\ pH \text{ units}$$

Therefore, the final *pH* will be:

$$7.26 - 0.17 = 7.09$$

If there was no oxyhemoglobin at all, the addition of 10 mmol of acid to 1000 mL of the solution would have decreased the *pH* of the solution to about 2.

The most abundant buffer of the body are the proteins of the cells and plasma, chiefly because of their very significant concentrations. The diffusion of the two elements of the bicarbonate buffer system (i.e., CO_2, and to a lesser extent HCO_3^-) through cell membranes causes the intracellular *pH* to change approximately in proportion to the extracellular *pH*. Thus, *all the intracellular buffer systems help buffer the extracellular fluid as well*. Experimental studies reveal that about three-quarters of all the chemical buffering capacity of the body fluids is inside the cells. Most of this is attributed to the buffering capacity of intracellular proteins. However, the slowness of the diffusion of H^+ and bicarbonate ions across the cell membranes (except for the red cells) often delays the function of the intracellular buffers to buffer extracellular acid-base abnormalities for many hours.

4.9.1 Bone as a Buffer

Bone also has buffering capacity. After an acid load, bone removes some of the excess H^+ in exchange for sodium and potassium, which results in bone demineralization and the release of buffer compounds $CaCO_3$ and $CaHPO_4$ into the extracellular fluid. Prolonged acidosis (e.g., in chronic renal failure) causes bone demineralization and *osteomalacia*.

Bone also plays an important role in withstanding a base load. As an example, augmented bone deposition of carbonate is developed after administration of sodium bicarbonate.

High-protein intake causes more acid load, and a consequent bone buffering activity which increases Ca^{2+} release and urinary Ca^{2+} excretion. This is the reason that a high-protein intake enhances the risk of calcium oxalate stone formation.

4.10 Renal Regulation of Extracellular Hydrogen Ion Concentration

The kidneys regulate the bicarbonate (HCO_3^-) concentration in two major ways:

1. variable reabsorption of the filtered bicarbonate at glomerulus, and
2. addition of new bicarbonate to the plasma.

These two mechanisms are totally inter-related and are achieved by a single process—tubular secretion of H^+. Examination of the reversible reaction:

$$H_2O + CO_2 \rightleftharpoons H^+ + HCO_3^- \tag{4.2}$$

makes it clear how regulation of the plasma bicarbonate concentration controls extracellular fluid hydrogen ion concentration. When plasma hydrogen ion concentration has been decreased (*alkalosis*), it can be returned to its normal value by reducing plasma bicarbonate concentration, thereby proceeding the reaction in Eq. (4.2) to the right and forming more hydrogen ions. The kidneys do this by failing to reabsorb all the filtered bicarbonate during alkalosis, permitting this unabsorbed bicarbonate to be excreted in the urine (an alkaline urine). In fact, the excretion of a bicarbonate ion in the urine has practically the same effect on the blood as would adding a hydrogen ion to the blood. This is *the renal compensation for alkalosis*.

Conversely, when plasma hydrogen ion concentration has been raised (*acidosis*), the kidney reabsorbs all the filtered bicarbonate, and in addition, new bicarbonate ions are created in renal tubular cells and liberated to the plasma, thereby augmenting the plasma bicarbonate concentration, and forcing the reaction in Eq. (4.2) to the left, lowering hydrogen ion concentration, and raising plasma *pH* toward normal. As will be seen later, the renal addition of new bicarbonate ion to the plasma is associated with the excretion of an equal amount of hydrogen ion in the urine (an acid urine). Therefore, the addition of new bicarbonate ion to the blood is essentially the same as the excretion of acid. Thus, "the kidney has added new bicarbonate ion to the blood" is synonymous to the statement, "kidney has excreted acid." This is *the renal compensation for acidosis*. Therefore, to compensate alkalosis, the kidneys excrete an alkaline urine and acidify the blood, and in response to acidosis, they excrete an acid urine and alkalinize the blood.

4.10.1 Bicarbonate Reabsorption

Bicarbonate is entirely filtered at the glomerulus, though in a normal condition, with no alkalosis, almost all is reabsorbed.

Example The normal plasma bicarbonate concentration is 24 mEq/L. Calculate the daily filtered bicarbonate in the kidneys, if the *glomerular filtration rate* (GFR) is 180 L/day.

Solution:

$$\begin{aligned}\text{Filtered } HCO_3^- /\text{day} &= GFR \times \left[HCO_3^-\right]_{\text{Plasma}}\\ &= 180 \times 24\\ &= 4320\,\text{mEq/day}\end{aligned}$$

This is about four times the total body buffering capacity. The failure to reabsorb this filtered bicarbonate is similar to adding more than 4 L of normal hydrochloric acid to the body, which is apparently catastrophic. Thus, *essentially no bicarbonate*

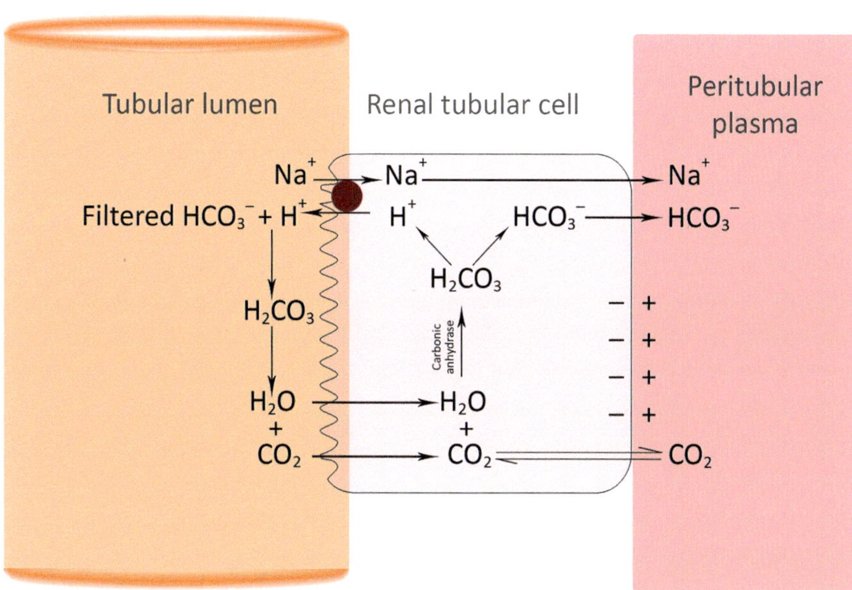

Fig. 4.11 Renal bicarbonate reabsorption

appears in the urine and all is reabsorbed normally. The reabsorption of bicarbonate is primarily active, and its passive reabsorption is negligible. The active mechanism by which the bicarbonate is reabsorbed comprises hydrogen ion secretion (Fig. 4.11).

The CO_2 in the peritubular plasma enters the renal tubular cells. There, it hydrates to make carbonic acid (H_2CO_3), a reaction which is catalyzed by intracellular carbonic anhydrase. The resultant carbonic acid then decomposes to hydrogen ion and bicarbonate. The bicarbonate moves into the interstitial fluid by simple diffusion down its electrochemical gradient (the intracellular space is negative relative to the interstitial fluid). Meanwhile, the hydrogen ion produced is secreted actively into the tubular lumen where it reacts with a filtered bicarbonate ion to produce carbonic acid, which dissociates to water and CO_2; these diffuse into the cell and then either diffuse into the peritubular plasma or are used in the reactions to create another hydrogen ion. Note that the bicarbonate ion in the peritubular plasma is not the one that was filtered. However, the net result is the same as if the same bicarbonate ion had been reabsorbed. It must also be noted that the hydrogen ion which was secreted into the lumen is in fact recycled; in effect, it is not excreted in the urine. Therefore, any secreted hydrogen ion (acid) that reacts with the luminal bicarbonate ion to reabsorb it does not influence the urinary acid excretion. Another point is that *the tubular secretion of hydrogen ion is coupled with sodium reabsorption* and consequently, the rate of bicarbonate reabsorption (H^+ secretion) is influenced by other mechanisms that regulate sodium reabsorption in the proximal tubule. As an example, volume expansion, which inhibits sodium reabsorption, decreases bicarbonate reabsorption, whereas volume contraction causes it to rise. The reabsorption of bicarbonate occurs throughout the nephron, with the exception of the descending loop of Henle. Besides this intracellular carbonic anhydrase, there are also some which are in the cell membrane of the proximal tubule luminal cells, which catalyze the intraluminal decomposition of the very large amount of carbonic acid formed in this part. For this reason, about 80%–90% of the filtered bicarbonate is reabsorbed in the proximal tubule; the remainder is usually reabsorbed by the loop of Henle and distal tubule.

4.10.2 Addition of New Bicarbonate to the Plasma and Renal Excretion of Acid

The renal compensation for acidosis is not only to reabsorb all the filtered bicarbonate but also to create new bicarbonate and acid excretion, so that the amount of bicarbonate in the renal veins exceeds that which entered the kidneys originally. The mechanism by which new bicarbonate is produced and added to the plasma is primarily the same as that for bicarbonate reabsorption, that is, tubular acid secretion (Fig. 4.12). The only difference between these two processes is that the secreted hydrogen ion, instead of combining with filtered bicarbonate (as in the case of bicarbonate reabsorption) reacts with other buffers in the lumen (or, to an extremely small degree, remains free in solution) and is excreted.

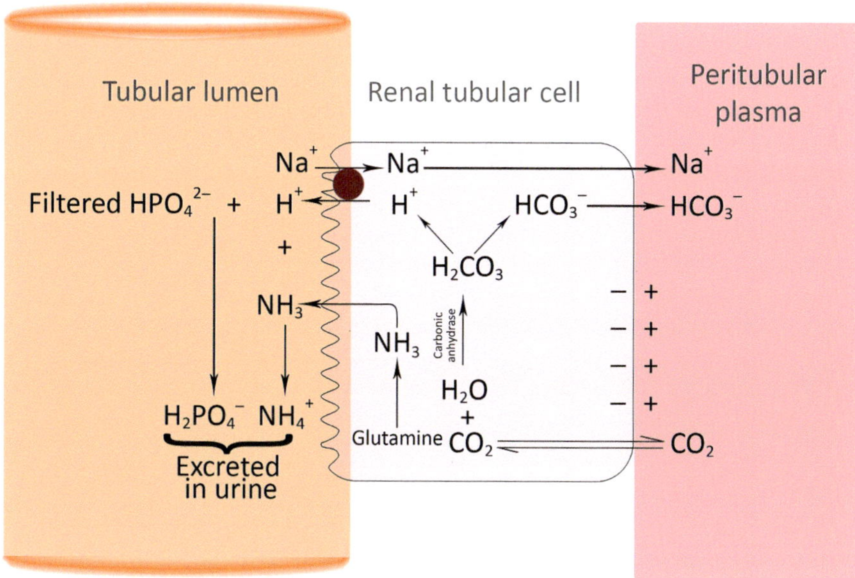

Fig. 4.12 Renal acid excretion and addition of new bicarbonate

As mentioned earlier, phosphate and ammonia are the two most important urinary buffers. Phosphate (HPO_4^{2-}) enters the lumen simply by glomerular filtration, but ammonia (NH_3), unlike phosphate, gains entry to the tubular lumen not by filtration, but rather by tubular synthesis (from glutamine) and secretion. Creatinine, organic acids, and other urinary buffers also participate in the formation of titratable acids and H^+ excretion, but their influence is negligible due to their very low concentration.

Clearly, the process of hydrogen ion secretion is the same tubular mechanism explained already, but the net overall result is different simply because the secreted acid reacts with phosphate or ammonia rather by filtered bicarbonate. Therefore, the bicarbonate created within the tubular cell and entering the plasma is a new bicarbonate which increases the plasma bicarbonate and alkalinizes it. It should be remarked that the addition of new bicarbonate to the blood by the kidneys is accompanied by the excretion of an equivalent amount of acid in the urine. In this case, in contrast to the bicarbonate reabsorption, the secreted hydrogen ion is trapped by urinary buffers and excreted in the urine (an acid urine). Thus, when kidneys add new bicarbonate to the blood, they are indeed excreting acid from the body, and alkalinizing it.

Example What happens to the renal acid secretion, if the arterial pCO_2 increases?

Solution: Carbon dioxide can freely penetrate through the cell membrane (by simple diffusion). Therefore, an increase in arterial pCO_2 causes an almost immediate equivalent increase in pCO_2 within the tubular cells. Reconsidering Fig. 4.12 and Le Chatelier's principle, an increase of intracellular pCO_2 provokes H_2CO_3 formation and results in an elevated intracellular hydrogen ion concentration. Subsequently, it is this change that directly increases the rate of tubular hydrogen ion (acid) secretion. Thus, *the ultimate stimulus for hydrogen ion secretion is not the* pCO_2 per se but rather the fall in intracellular *pH* it induces.

Cell membrane is less permeable to the diffusion of H^+. Therefore, the change in intracellular *pH* is much less dependent upon changes in extracellular and blood *pH*. Accordingly, the rate of renal acid secretion correlates better with pCO_2 than with blood *pH*. Three other mechanisms which augment the rate of renal hydrogen ion excretion include:

1. increased sodium concentration in the distal renal tubule,
2. hypokalemia, which causes a decline in intracellular *pH*, and
3. acidosis, which stimulates ammonia synthesis in the renal tubular cells.

Contrarily, low sodium concentration in distal nephron, hypoaldosteronism, or alkalosis reduces renal acid excretion.

Example Write the Henderson-Hasselbalch equation for the ammonia-ammonium system. What is the ratio $[NH_3]/[NH_4^+]$ at normal *pH* of 7.4 or less?

Solution:

$$\underset{\text{Conjugate acid}}{NH_4^+} \rightleftharpoons H^+ + \underset{\text{Conjugate base}}{NH_3}$$

and

$$pH = pK + \log\frac{[\text{Conjugate base}]}{[\text{Conjugate acid}]}$$

Then:

$$pH = 9.25 + \log\frac{[NH_3]}{[NH_4^+]}$$

At the *pH* 7.4, we have:

$$7.4 = 9.25 + \log\frac{[NH_3]}{[NH_4^+]}$$

Therefore:

$$-1.85 = \log\frac{[NH_3]}{[NH_4^+]}$$

and

$$\frac{[NH_3]}{[NH_4^+]} = 10^{-1.85}$$

$$= 0.01$$

This suggests that, given the normal *pH* of 7.4 or less, almost all NH_3 that enters the tubular lumen will at once pick up hydrogen ions to form NH_4^+. Therefore, as long as a supply of NH_3 is accessible, H^+ secretion and the net addition of bicarbonate to the blood can proceed with no danger of reaching the minimum achievable urinary *pH* of 4.4.

In some situations, certain organic compounds may appear in the tubular fluid in a sufficient quantity to permit them to act also as important buffers. An interesting example is a patient with *diabetic ketoacidosis* (DKA). As a result of insulin deficiency, the patient develops acidosis because of the formation of the large quantity of acetoacetic and β-hydroxybutyric acid, which at plasma *pH* completely ionize to generate anions (acetoacetate and β-hydroxybutyrate) and hydrogen ion. These anions are filtered at the glomerulus but are just partially reabsorbed. They are accessible in the tubular fluid to buffer only a fraction of the hydrogen ions secreted by the tubules, to compensate for the acidosis.

What you have seen in this chapter was a bird's eye view of what happens in a normal person. In the next chapters, you will discover the pathologic conditions of the acid-base chemistry in more detail.

4.11 Things to Remember

Ventilation, Perfusion, and Gas Exchange

In an upright position, basal ventilation and perfusion per unit volume of lung tissue exceed those of the apices. The $\dot{V}/\dot{Q}$ ratio increases from 0.6 at the base to about 3.3 at the apex; thus, apical alveoli are grossly overventilated, whereas basilar ones are overperfused.

Most gas exchange occurs in the lower part of the lungs. $\dot{V}/\dot{Q}$ mismatch is responsible for many hypoxic states. CO_2 penetration through the blood-gas interface is 20 times more than that of O_2.

The respiratory quotient is defined as:

$$R = \frac{\text{Rate of } CO_2 \text{ output}}{\text{Rate of } O_2 \text{ uptake}}$$

and, typically, its average value is 0.8.

The alveolar oxygen tension is:

$$p_A O_2 = f_i O_2 (p_B - 47) - \frac{p_a CO_2}{0.8}$$

The alveoli-arterial oxygen tension difference is usually the result of $\dot{V}/\dot{Q}$ mismatch and averages 8 mm Hg in normal young persons and increases linearly with age.

Hemoglobin and Transfer of Oxygen

Oxygenation of hemoglobin is not an oxidation reaction. The hemoglobin whose iron is oxidized is incapable of carrying oxygen and is called methemoglobin.

Oxygen is carried to the tissues in two ways—bounded with hemoglobin and as dissolved oxygen, therefore:

$$O_2\ \text{Content} = 1.34\left[Hb\right]\frac{Hb_{\text{Sat\%}}}{100} + 0.003\ p_{\text{a}}O_2$$

Oxyhemoglobin Dissociation Curve

In the periphery, the oxyhemoglobin dissociation curve shifts to the right due to increased temperature, pCO_2, red cell organic phosphate, and decreased *pH*. Consequently, the affinity of hemoglobin for O_2 decreases, and oxygen is delivered to the tissues.

Carriage of Carbon Dioxide

Carbon dioxide is carried by the blood in three forms:

1. as dissolved CO_2 in plasma,
2. combined with hemoglobin, and
3. as bicarbonate.

Control of Respiration

The neural centers controlling the respiration are mostly placed in the reticular formation of medulla oblongata. They are extremely sensitive to arterial pCO_2 and regulate its level by changing the rate and depth of respiration.

The carotid body and aortic arch chemoreceptors are stimulated mainly by hypoxia and, to a lesser extent, by hypercapnia. The carotid body is also sensitive to acidemia. The afferent signals are carried to the medulla by the glossopharyngeal (IX) and vagus (X) nerves.

Buffers

Buffers are the first line of defense of living organisms against variations in their internal *pH*. The intracellular buffers help buffer the extracellular fluid as well. Proteins are the most abundant buffers in the body. Much of the buffering activity of oxyhemoglobin in the physiologic range is done by imidazole groups. The most important buffers of intracellular space are proteins and phosphate. The most important buffer of plasma and extracellular fluid is carbonic acid-bicarbonate conjugate pair. The most important buffers of the urinary system are phosphate and ammonia. Bone can buffer acid and alkali load. Prolonged acidosis leads to bone demineralization and osteomalacia.

Renal Regulation of $[H^+]$

The kidneys regulate the bicarbonate HCO_3^- concentration in two major ways:

1. variable reabsorption of the filtered bicarbonate at glomerulus, and
2. addition of new bicarbonate to the plasma.

The mechanisms of bicarbonate reabsorption and acid secretion are essentially the same, i.e., tubular acid secretion. "The kidney has added new bicarbonate ion to the blood" is synonymous to the statement "kidney has excreted acid." Essentially no bicarbonate appears in the urine and all is reabsorbed normally.

The stimulus for tubular hydrogen ion secretion is decreased intracellular *pH*. Conditions which decrease intracellular *pH* (i.e., increased renal acid excretion) include hypercapnia, increased $[Na^+]$ in distal nephron, hypokalemia, and acidosis.

Henderson-Hasselbalch Equation

Based on what was mentioned, respiratory system and kidneys control the p_aCO_2 and serum $[H^+]$, respectively. Therefore, the Henderson-Hasselbalch equation (Eq. (3.5)) can be rewritten in its mnemonic form:

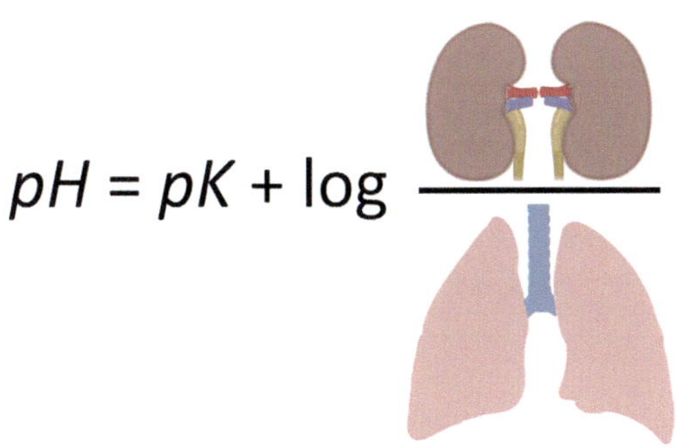

References

1. West JB. Respiratory physiology. 9th ed. Philadelphia: Lippincott Williams and Wilkins; 2012.
2. Cox MM, Nelson DL. Lehninger principles of biochemistry. 6th ed. New York: W. H. Freeman; 2012.
3. Perutz MF. Nature of haem-haem interaction. Nature. 1972;237(5357):495–9. https://doi.org/10.1038/237495a0.
4. Benner A, Patel AK, Singh K, Dua A. Physiology, Bohr effect. Treasure Island, FL: StatPearls; 2020.
5. Drechsler M, Morris J. Carbon dioxide narcosis. Treasure Island, FL: StatPearls; 2020.
6. Rudrappa M, Modi P, Bollu PC. Cheyne stokes respirations. Treasure Island, FL: StatPearls; 2020.
7. Coniglio AC, Mentz RJ. Sleep breathing disorders in heart failure. Heart Fail Clin. 2020;16(1):45–51. https://doi.org/10.1016/j.hfc.2019.08.009.

Introduction to Acid-Base Chemistry and Arterial Blood Gases

5

In the preceding section, the physiologic basis of acid-base chemistry was reviewed. In this chapter, the basic clinical viewpoints, including terminology and an introductory approach to a patient with a suspected acid-base disorder, will be described.

5.1 Terminology

The nomenclature of acid-base chemistry and arterial blood gas (ABG) analysis is very easy to understand if one re-examines the well-known Henderson-Hasselbalch equation (Eq. (3.5)), which correlates blood *pH*, pCO_2, and $\left[HCO_3^-\right]$.

$$\left.\begin{matrix}\text{Alkalemia}\uparrow\\ \text{Acidemia}\downarrow\end{matrix}\right\} pH = pK + \log\frac{\left[HCO_3^-\right]\left.\begin{Bmatrix}\uparrow\text{Alkalosis}\\ \downarrow\text{Acidosis}\end{Bmatrix}\right\}\text{Metabolic}}{\alpha\, pCO_2\left.\begin{Bmatrix}\uparrow\text{Acidosis}\\ \downarrow\text{Alkalosis}\end{Bmatrix}\right\}\text{Respiratory}}$$

Acidemia refers to any condition with a detectable decrease in blood *pH*, whereas *alkalemia* means an increased blood *pH*. Therefore, acidemia and alkalemia just describe the blood *pH*.

Accumulation of acids in the blood or the depletion of body alkaline reserve (bicarbonate content) creates a condition, the so-called *acidosis*. On the other hand, *alkalosis* is a pathologic state resulting from the collection of base, or loss of acid (without a proportionate loss of base) in the body fluids. Thus, the terms acidosis and alkalosis only describe the underlying pathologic process that tends to change the blood *pH*. In most conditions, an acidotic process (acidosis) leads to acidemia and an alkalotic process (alkalosis) to alkalemia. However, this may not be true in patients with mixed acid-base disturbances in whom the final blood *pH* depends upon the balance between the different concomitant disorders.

F. Habibzadeh et al., *Pathophysiologic Basis of Acid-Base Disorders*,
https://doi.org/10.1007/978-981-16-0526-0_5

5.2 Bedside Approach to a Patient with a Suspected Acid-Base Disorder

Before any decision has been made, at first a complete history, including history of previous medication (e.g., acetazolamide, thiazide, salicylic acid, etc.), ingestion of toxic agents (e.g., methanol, ethanol, ethylene glycol, etc.) or therapeutic measures (e.g., mechanical ventilation, nasogastric suction, hyperalimentation, etc.) should be taken. The most notable clinical settings which may be associated with an acid-base disturbance consist of vomiting, renal disease, chronic bronchitis, emphysema, pneumothorax, asthma, pulmonary edema, uncontrolled diabetes mellitus, ureteral diversion, cystic fibrosis, and biliary-pancreatic fistula. Thereby, the past medical history of such problems may be helpful.

In the second step, a careful physical examination should be performed. Special attention should be paid to the vital signs (temperature, pulse rate, respiratory rate, and blood pressure) and general appearance of the patient. They may give you important information about the condition of the patient. A rapid pulse (tachycardia) or hypotension demonstrates a low cardiac output and its consequent acid-base derangement. A deep rapid respiration or a shallow slow breathing, reflect hyper- or hypo-ventilation, respectively, and may be a clue for an underlying acid-base disorder.

The following are the most important points which should be noted in the physical examination:

General appearance: Pallor, cyanosis, restlessness, jaundice, and edema

Head and neck: Airway and any possibility of its obstruction, neck veins and jugular venous pressure (JVP), thyroid size, and tracheal deviation

Chest: Rales, wheeze, decreased breathing sound, and structural abnormality such as scoliosis

Heart: Cardiac murmurs, which may be a clue for a low cardiac output state such as aortic stenosis (AS) or aortic insufficiency (AI), and shunting of blood through a ventricular septal defect (VSD), atrial septal defect (ASD), or patent ductus arteriosus (PDA)

Abdomen: Possibility of ascites, organomegaly, collateral veins, paradoxical motion of the abdomen, edema, and muscular weakness

Extremities: Coldness, cyanosis of nail beds, and edema

Finally, serum electrolyte (Na^+, K^+, Cl^-) concentrations should be measured. As a general rule, any patient with a suspected acid-base derangement should be investigated for any arterial blood gas or serum electrolyte imbalances prior to the initiation of any treatment [1].

The serum potassium concentration ($[K^+]$) is often helpful, especially in conjunction with the blood *pH*. Serum $[K^+]$ can be altered by primary acid-base disturbances. When serum $[H^+]$ is higher than normal (acidemia), extracellular H^+ is exchanged with intracellular K^+; thus, the serum $[K^+]$ will be increased. As a general rule, the plasma potassium concentration is raised by 0.6 mEq/L for each 0.1 unit decrease in arterial *pH*, that is:

$$\Delta\left[K^{+}\right] = -6\Delta pH \quad (5.1)$$

The negative sign indicates that the directions of variations are opposite, that is, a decrease in *pH* causes an increase in serum [K^+].

Example The plasma [K^+] and *pH* of a patient with diabetic ketoacidosis (DKA) are 4 mEq/L and 7.1, respectively. What will be the serum potassium concentration if the *pH* is corrected to 7.4?

Solution: $\Delta\left[K^{+}\right] = -6\Delta pH$

The *pH* change is 0.3 (= 7.4–7.1), therefore:

$$\begin{aligned}\Delta\left[K^{+}\right] &= -6 \times 0.3 \\ &= -1.8\,\mathrm{mEq/L}\end{aligned}$$

Thus, serum [K^+] will be decreased to 2.2 (= 4–1.8) mEq/L, a life-threatening value, which requires prompt therapeutic measures. Therefore, *the correction of acidemia in a patient with hypokalemia, or even lower limit of normokalemia, without administration of potassium salts, may lead to a severe hypokalemic state and even death.*

The study of changes of serum bicarbonate level $\left(\left[HCO_3^-\right]\right)$ comprises one of the major debates and will be explored in detail in the following chapters.

Other laboratory evaluations, useful in the approach to acid-base imbalance, include blood sugar (e.g., in diabetic ketoacidosis), blood urea nitrogen (BUN; e.g., in renal failure), blood culture (e.g., in sepsis), and hemoglobin concentration. Also, a chest roentgenogram may be helpful in those with pulmonary disease.

5.3 Indications for Arterial Blood Gas Analysis

Arterial blood gas analysis is recommended whenever the patient is suspected to have either an acid-base disorder (e.g., chronic renal failure, diabetic ketoacidosis, diarrhea, septicemia) or gas exchange impairment (e.g., chronic bronchitis, emphysema, pulmonary edema, atelectasis).

5.4 Obtaining the Sample

An arterial blood sample can be obtained either by an arterial puncture or via an indwelling arterial line. A glass syringe is preferred, since it does not allow the gases to be exchanged, and should be washed with heparin solution so that it fills and empties freely. Only adequate heparin is utilized to fill the tip of the syringe and the needle. *Excess heparin dilutes the estimated hemoglobin concentration, and its extra acidity reduces the real pH*. Air bubbles, even small ones, must be expelled from the syringe, thus avoiding faults in the measurement of pO_2 and pCO_2 caused by gas equilibration with the bubble. After sampling, the syringe should be capped and entirely rotated to let the blood mix with heparin. Then, the sample should be carried to the analyzer in ice and under anaerobic condition. The analysis must be done as soon as possible because delay, especially when the leukocyte count is high, can markedly decrease the pO_2 due to cellular oxygen consumption. A plastic syringe can be employed satisfactorily and gives precise values, when skilled staff obtain blood and analysis is done promptly.

It is important to report the temperature and hemoglobin concentration of the patient. Also the oxygen fraction of the inspired air (f_iO_2), and the time of sampling should be given in the requisition sheet.

The best site for arterial puncture is the radial artery. If the radial artery is used, the patency of the ulnar artery must be proved by means of an *Allen's test* [2, 3].

5.4.1 Allen's Test

If there is no ample flow in the ulnar artery, we should not puncture the radial artery because it may cause serious damage to the hand circulation. To check if ulnar artery has enough blood flow, we need to perform the Allen's test. To do so, occlude both radial and ulnar arteries of the patient at the wrist by applying pressure over them, while he or she makes a tight fist. The patient should open his hand. While keeping pressure on the radial artery, release the ulnar artery. If the ulnar artery is open and its circulation is sufficient, the hand should flush red within 5–10 s. A radial puncture can then be done safely [2]. If the hand remains pale or the color return is delayed, do not perform the arterial puncture as incompetent collateral circulation is present. It is better to select an alternate site.

The next sites for an arterial puncture are the brachial artery; if this is not approachable, the femoral artery. In infants, the temporal artery is an appropriate location for arterial blood sampling. Intra-arterial catheters promote blood withdrawal, particularly when blood gas analysis should be examined frequently (more than five samples per day), and are usually placed in the radial artery. In such conditions, a continuous flushing system with a low dose of heparin is utilized to sustain the patency of the line.

5.4.2 Complications of Arterial Puncture and Cannulation

The most significant complications of arterial puncture and cannulation are hematoma, bleeding, arterial thrombosis, arterial occlusion (which may lead to compartment syndrome), local infection, and sepsis.

5.5 Analysis of the Sample

The most widely used analyzers are equipped with electrodes for measuring *pH*, pCO_2, and pO_2. The bicarbonate concentration is then obtained either from a nomogram or calculated by a built-in preprogrammed calculator.

5.6 Venous Blood Gas Analysis

Venous blood is easier to take and is expected to be as correct as the arterial blood for gas analysis [4]. However, central or peripheral venous blood gas analysis can be done only as a crude estimate for evaluation of acid-base status in critically ill patients. An arterial or venous pCO_2 of 80–100 mm Hg means a clinically significant hypoventilation, and an arterial or venous pO_2 below 35 mm Hg, in any case, reflects tissue hypoxia.

Venous blood pO_2 equilibrates with tissue oxygen pressure; thus, it can indicate the tissue oxygenation. Patients with circulatory failure, despite a normal or even an elevated arterial oxygen tension, may develop a low central or peripheral venous pO_2 which discloses tissue hypoxia.

In general, the venous *pH* is 0.03–0.05 units lower than that of the arterial, and venous bicarbonate concentration and pCO_2 are 1–3 mEq/L and 5–7 mm Hg more than those of the arterial, respectively.

5.7 Anion Gap

Routine laboratory examinations can give us a measure of serum concentrations of some anions (Cl^-, HCO_3^-) and cations (Na^+, K^+, Ca^{2+}, Mg^{2+}), but, there are some anions (e.g., lactate) whose serum levels change in certain conditions. As there is a balance between the quantity of cations and anions in the plasma, the amount of these *unmeasurable anions* can be found by subtracting the amounts of measurable anions from that of the measurable cations. The amount of unmeasurable anions is called the *anion gap* (*AG*) [5].

$$AG = [\text{measurable cations}] - [\text{measurable anions}]$$
$$= \left([Na^+] + [K^+] + [Ca^{2+}] + [Mg^{2+}]\right) - \left([Cl^-] + [HCO_3^-]\right)$$

Except for Na^+, other cations which are present in the plasma (i.e., K^+, Ca^{2+}, Mg^{2+}) have little or no effect on health or disease; thus, they may be excluded from the above formula; the *AG* can then be calculated as:

$$AG = [Na^+] - \left([Cl^-] + [HCO_3^-]\right) \tag{5.2}$$

In this way, its normal range is about 12 ± 2 mEq/L.

Example What is the *AG* in a normal person, with a serum electrolyte composition of $[Na^+]$ = 140 mEq/L, $[Cl^-]$ = 105 mEq/L, $\left[HCO_3^-\right]$ = 25 mEq/L.

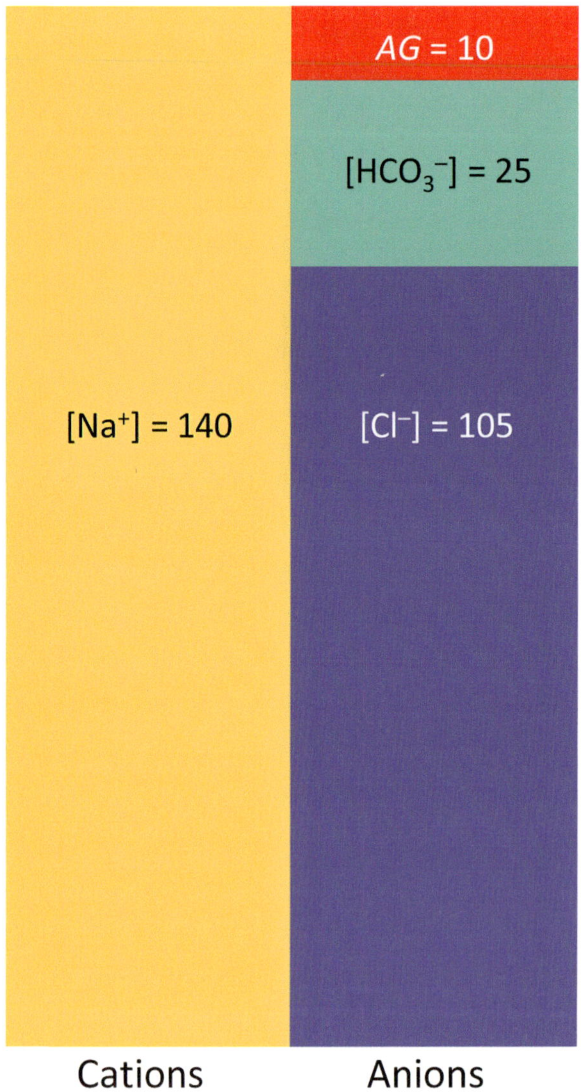

Solution:

$$
\begin{aligned}
AG &= \left[Na^+\right] - \left(\left[Cl^-\right] + \left[HCO_3^-\right]\right) \\
&= 140 - (105 + 25) \\
&= 10\,\text{mEq}/\text{L}
\end{aligned}
$$

which is normal.

Example Determine the AG in a patient with acute renal failure, and serum electrolyte profile of $[Na^+] = 140$ mEq/L, $[Cl^-] = 105$ mEq/L, $\left[HCO_3^-\right] = 12$ mEq/L.

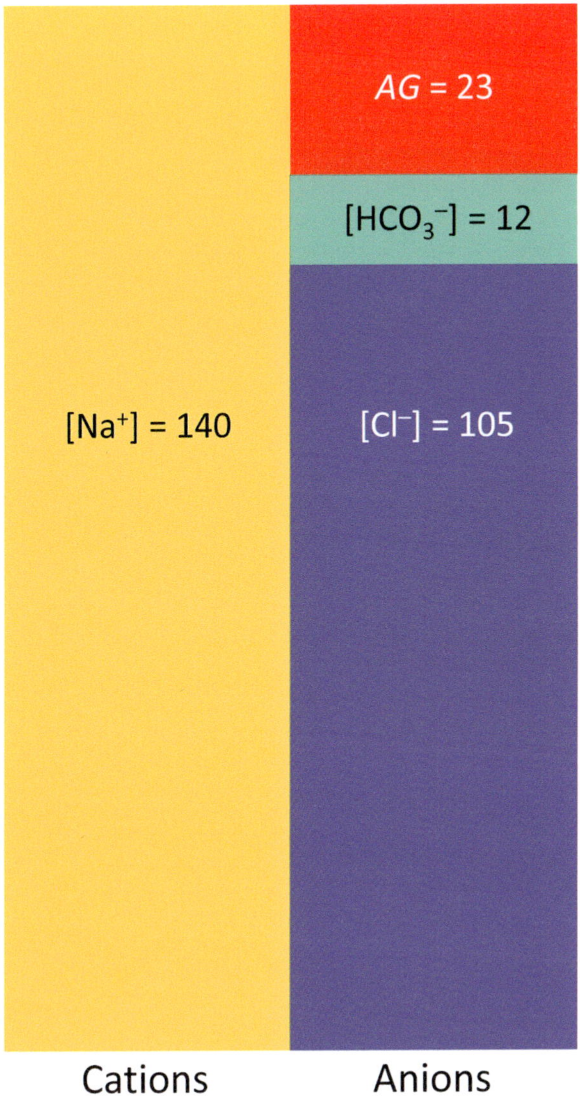

Solution:

$$\begin{aligned} AG &= \left[Na^+\right] - \left(\left[Cl^-\right] + \left[HCO_3^-\right]\right) \\ &= 140 - (105 + 12) \\ &= 23\,\text{mEq/L} \end{aligned}$$

which is more than 12 mEq/L.

An increased *AG* usually indicates the accumulation of acid in body fluids. This condition is known as *high-anion gap acidosis*. In such cases, the added hydrogen ions (which are equal to the added anions) are buffered by plasma bicarbonate. Thus, for each mEq/L increase in the *AG* there should be an equal decrease in the plasma $\left[HCO_3^-\right]$, and therefore, a consequent raise in the *AG* will be ensued. The only exception in strong acids is hydrochloric acid (HCl). The addition of its anion (Cl^-), which is measurable, counterbalances the effect of the reduced bicarbonate concentration and causes no net change in the *AG*. *An AG greater than 25 mEq/L is only seen in diabetic ketoacidosis (DKA), lactic acidosis, or poisoning with methanol, ethylene glycol, or salicylate*. The patient with a high *AG* seems to be more ill and has a higher admission and mortality rates. In those disorders which are associated with an accumulation of cationic proteins (e.g., myeloma) the *AG* may be reduced [5, 6].

5.8 Base Excess (BE)

If some alkali presents in the blood, the *pH* is increased and can be restored to 7.4 (normal *pH*) by the addition of some acid to the blood (i.e., titration). The added H^+ ions combine with excess hydroxyl ions. Some are spent in furnishing the blood buffers, which lose their power as a result of surplus OH^-, and others cause the *pH* to return to normal. After completion of the procedure (by the time the *pH* has reached 7.4), the amount of added acid can be used as an estimate for the concentration of the excess alkali in the original blood. If this process is performed at 37 °C and at a pCO_2 of 40 mm Hg, the concentration of excess base presented in the primary blood sample is called *base excess* (BE) [7, 8].

In the same way, extra acid in the blood decreases the *pH*. The *pH* may be returned to 7.4 by neutralizing the excess H^+ by adding some alkali (e.g., NaOH). If the procedure is carried out at 37 °C and at a pCO_2 of 40 mm Hg, the measure of the base utilized can help us to find out the concentration of the excess acid which existed in the initial blood. This concentration is termed *base deficit* or negative base excess (BE).

A positive BE suggests an excess of base, whereas a negative BE (base deficit) means an excess of non-volatile (non-carbonic, fixed) acid or a deficiency of bicarbonate. In other words, *BE is a measure of the net metabolic component of the acid-base disturbance*. This metabolic disturbance may be due to either a primary cause or a secondary compensatory mechanism for a respiratory acid-base disorder.

5.9 Normal Values

Table 5.1 shows the normal laboratory values for arterial and venous blood.

Table 5.1 Normal values for arterial and venous blood

Parameters	Arterial	Venous
pH	7.35 to 7.45	7.32 to 7.42
pCO_2 (mm Hg)	35 to 45	41 to 51
$\left[HCO_3^-\right]$ (mEq/L)	22 to 26	24 to 28
Base excess (mEq/L)	−2 to +2	
pO_2 (mm Hg)		
Adult	80 to100	
Over age 65	75 to 85	36 to 44
Newborn	60 to 70	
O_2 percentage saturation	96 to 97	40 to 70
O_2 content (mL/dL blood)		
Men	17.5 to 23.0	
Women	16.0 to 21.5	

5.10 Bicarbonate Space

Treatment of some acid-base disorders may include intravenous infusion of alkali or acid. Administration of such substances without any knowledge of the *bicarbonate space of distribution*, which from now on will simply be called bicarbonate space, is impossible. Bicarbonate space (in liters) is approximately 50% of the body weight (in kilograms), that is

$$\text{Bicarbonate space}_{\text{L}} = 0.5Wt_{\text{kg}} \tag{5.3}$$

This quantity is really the volume of distribution of bicarbonate, the available body fluid volume in which bicarbonate can be penetrated and distributed. For more clarity, it is better to give an example.

Example What is the total bicarbonate content in a 35-year-old man with a body weight of 70 kg and a serum $\left[HCO_3^-\right]$ of 25 mEq/L?

Solution: The volume of distribution of bicarbonate or bicarbonate space can be simply calculated as:

$$\begin{aligned}\text{Bicarbonate space}_{\text{L}} &= 0.5Wt_{\text{kg}}\\ &= 0.5\times 70\\ &= 35\,\text{L}\end{aligned}$$

Considering the definition of bicarbonate space, the bicarbonate content, which is the total amount of bicarbonate in body, can then be found by a simple multiplication:

$$\begin{aligned}\text{Bicarbonate content}_{\text{mEq/L}} &= \text{Bicarbonate space}_{\text{L}} \times \left[\text{HCO}_3^-\right]_{\text{mEq/L}} \\ &= 35 \times 25 \\ &= 875\,\text{mEq}\end{aligned}$$

5.11 Systemic Effects of Acidemia

Blood *pH* lower than 7.2 enhances epinephrine release, which applies a positive inotropic effect. Thus, the heart rate and the cardiac output are augmented. A greater decline in *pH* (<7.1) dampens cardiac muscle contraction. This effect is exerted in various ways; *acidemia suppresses the influence of catecholamine and calcium on the heart*. Moreover, it provokes the accumulation of acetylcholine through the blockade of cholinesterase. As a result, the heart rate falls, cardiac output diminishes, and the patient may develop heart failure and even pulmonary edema. The clinical picture depends on the algebraic sum of the acidemia-induced positive and negative inotropic effects. The positive inotropic effects of acidemia are abolished in those who receive calcium channel or β-adrenergic blocker agents. Therefore, they are more sensitive to the inhibitory effects of acidemia. Severe acidemia causes arteriolar dilation, venoconstriction and hypotension which is manifested as warm, well-perfused peripheral tissues, a condition which is known as *warm shock*.

Very low *pH* stimulates emesis. The patient vomits, and after loss of some gastric acid, transiently survives the life-threatening acidemia. Elevated hydrogen ion concentration also shifts the oxyhemoglobin dissociation curve to the right, thereby, enhancing tissue oxygenation. It also causes leukocytosis, with a count occasionally reaching 30 000–60 000/μL.

Prolonged acidosis causes osteomalacia; it results in mobilization of calcium and phosphate from the bone matrix, and depletion of bone minerals and, on the other hand, suppresses the conversion of 25-hydroxy cholecalciferol to 1,25-dihydroxy cholecalciferol (the active form of vitamin D), and interruption of calcium absorption in the gastrointestinal tract.

5.12 Systemic Effects of Alkalemia

The most common symptoms of alkalemia are central nervous system (CNS) manifestations which are secondary to the decreased cerebral blood flow and include confusion, obtundation, delirium, and decreased seizure threshold. A high *pH* also leads to a decrease in ionized calcium levels as a consequence of increased protein binding. This is why positive *Chvostek's* and *Trousseau's* signs may be present in alkalemic states [9]. Increased acetylcholine release and low serum ionized calcium concentration elevates muscular excitability; thus, in severe alkalemia ($pH > 7.55$) tetany may occur.

Alkalemia shifts the oxyhemoglobin dissociation curve to the left, thereby diminishing oxygen delivery to tissues and causing hypoxia. In addition, in alkalemia, extracellular potassium shifts into the cell and renal reabsorption of K^+ is decreased; thus, hypokalemia may ensue. Both hypoxia and hypokalemia disturb electrical stability and different cardiac arrhythmias may occur. Other cardiac complications of alkalemia include myocardial necrosis, increased sensitivity to cardiac glycosides (e.g., digoxin), reduced cardiac output, and a consequent hypotension.

Finally, and most importantly, because *alkalemia has a higher mortality than acidemia*, it should be carefully diagnosed and treated.

5.13 Things to Remember

Terminology is not difficult, if we look at the following equation carefully:

$$\left.\begin{matrix}\text{Alkalemia}\uparrow\\ \text{Acidemia}\downarrow\end{matrix}\right\} pH = pK + \log\frac{\left[HCO_3^-\right]\left\{\begin{matrix}\uparrow\text{Alkalosis}\\ \downarrow\text{Acidosis}\end{matrix}\right\}\text{Metabolic}}{\alpha\, pCO_2\left\{\begin{matrix}\uparrow\text{Acidosis}\\ \downarrow\text{Alkalosis}\end{matrix}\right\}\text{Respiratory}}$$

In a patient with suspected acid-base abnormalities, three steps should be taken sequentially.

1. Take a complete history.
2. Perform a careful physical examination.
3. Do laboratory examination (e.g., measurement of serum $[Na^+]$, $[K^+]$, $[Cl^-]$, blood sugar, blood urea, arterial blood gas analysis), and chest roentgenography.

Before the radial artery puncture is performed, the patency of the ulnar artery must be proved by means of an Allen's test. To achieve an accurate result, only adequate heparin should be used and air bubbles, even small ones, must be expelled from the syringe.

Serum potassium concentration usually alters as a consequence of the primary acid-base disturbances, that is:

$$\Delta\left[K^+\right] = -6\Delta pH$$

Thus, correction of acidemia in a patient with hypokalemia, or even a lower limit of normokalemia, without potassium administration, may lead to severe hypokalemia and even death.

The anion gap (*AG*) reflects the value of unmeasurable anions and is calculated as:

$$AG = \left[Na^+\right] - \left(\left[Cl^-\right] + \left[HCO_3^-\right]\right)$$

In this way, its normal range is 12 ± 2 mEq/L.

A positive base excess (BE) suggests an excess of base, whereas a negative BE (base deficit) means either an excess of non-volatile (non-carbonic, fixed) acid or a deficiency of bicarbonate. In other words, BE is a measure of net metabolic component of the acid-base disturbance. This metabolic disturbance may be either due to a primary cause, or a secondary compensatory mechanism for a respiratory acid-base disorder.

Bicarbonate space (in liters) is approximately 50% of the body weight (in kilograms), that is

$$\text{Bicarbonate space}_{\text{L}} = 0.5\, Wt_{\text{kg}}$$

References

1. Shrimanker I, Bhattarai S. Electrolytes. Treasure Island, FL: StatPearls; 2020.
2. Puttarajappa C, Rajan DS. Allen's test. N Engl J Med. 2010;363:e20. https://doi.org/10.1056/NEJMicm1001091.
3. Habib J, Baetz L, Satiani B. Assessment of collateral circulation to the hand prior to radial artery harvest. Vasc Med. 2012;17(5):352–61. https://doi.org/10.1177/1358863X12451514.
4. Rieser TM. Arterial and venous blood gas analyses. Top Companion Anim Med. 2013;28(3):86–90. https://doi.org/10.1053/j.tcam.2013.04.002.
5. Kraut JA, Nagami GT. The serum anion gap in the evaluation of acid-base disorders: what are its limitations and can its effectiveness be improved? Clin J Am Soc Nephrol. 2013;8(11):2018–24. https://doi.org/10.2215/CJN.04040413.
6. Jurado RL, del Rio C, Nassar G, Navarette J, Pimentel JL Jr. Low anion gap. South Med J. 1998;91(7):624–9. https://doi.org/10.1097/00007611-199807000-00004.
7. Berend K. Diagnostic use of base excess in acid-base disorders. N Engl J Med. 2018;378(15):1419–28. https://doi.org/10.1056/NEJMra1711860.
8. Juern J, Khatri V, Weigelt J. Base excess: a review. J Trauma Acute Care Surg. 2012;73(1):27–32. https://doi.org/10.1097/TA.0b013e318256999d.
9. Juan D. Hypocalcemia. Differential diagnosis and mechanisms. Arch Intern Med. 1979;139(10):1166–71. https://doi.org/10.1001/archinte.139.10.1166.

6 Respiratory Acidosis and Alkalosis

Definition Based on the foregoing discussions, it is clear that any factor that decreases pulmonary ventilation leads to the retention of carbon dioxide and subsequently increases arterial pCO_2 (hypercapnia). Considering the following reaction:

$$H_2O + CO_2 \rightleftharpoons H_2CO_3 \rightleftharpoons H^+ + HCO_3^-$$

and employing Le Chatelier's principle, a raised CO_2 concentration proceeds the above equation to the right and, ultimately, causes an increase in hydrogen ion concentrations, which in turn results in an acidosis. Since the pCO_2 is regulated by respiration, this type of acidosis, which is a consequence of a primary change in pCO_2, is termed *respiratory acidosis* [1].

Contrary to this, excessive pulmonary ventilation inverts the above process; CO_2 is removed from the blood and thus the arterial pCO_2 is reduced. The above reaction shifts to the left, and a resultant drop in plasma $[H^+]$ occurs. The reduction in serum $[H^+]$ leads to alkalosis, and, because this condition is a result of a primary alteration in pCO_2, it is called *respiratory alkalosis* [2]. The variation in serum $[H^+]$ in respiratory acidosis or alkalosis produces *acidemia* (a decrease in blood *pH*) or *alkalemia* (an increase in blood *pH*), respectively.

6.1 Causes of Respiratory Acidosis and Alkalosis

A person can induce respiratory acidosis in himself by simply holding his breath, which he can do until the *pH* of the body fluids drops to as low as possibly 7. On the other hand, he can voluntarily overbreathe and cause respiratory alkalosis up to the *pH* rise to around 7.9. Respiratory alkalosis can also physiologically occur in those who climb to high altitudes; the ambient air low oxygen content stimulates respiration; this, in turn, leads to excess loss of carbon dioxide and the subsequent generation of a mild respiratory alkalosis.

F. Habibzadeh et al., *Pathophysiologic Basis of Acid-Base Disorders*,
https://doi.org/10.1007/978-981-16-0526-0_6

A common cause of acute respiratory acidosis is sudden obstruction of the airways, e.g., secondary to foreign body aspiration, bronchospasm, or laryngospasm. However, any condition causing respiratory muscle malfunction, neuromuscular diseases affecting respiratory muscles, suppression of medullary respiratory centers (either by cerebral illness or drugs), cardiopulmonary arrest, or an abrupt fall in alveolar gas exchange may be accompanied by an acute respiratory acidosis and its outcomes [1, 3].

Chronic respiratory acidosis is more common in chronic lung diseases such as emphysema and chronic bronchitis, in which ventilation-perfusion mismatch presents and effective alveolar ventilation is reduced. Extreme obesity (BMI ≥ 35 kg/m^2) hampers the respiratory motions of the chest wall. This would restrict the flow of gas into and out of the alveolar space and in combination with the blunted chemoreflex to CO_2 leads to obesity hypoventilation syndrome (*Pickwickian* syndrome), which is characterized by chronic respiratory acidosis [4].

Common causes of respiratory alkalosis are central nervous system (CNS) lesions in the proximity of the medullary respiratory centers that either augment the stimulatory inputs or interfere with inhibitory impulses. Anxiety and hysteria, both of which indirectly induce hyperventilation via cortical pathways, are also important etiologies of acute respiratory alkalosis [2, 5]. Those pulmonary disorders which are associated with interference with alveolar gas exchange, such as chronic pulmonary fibrosis, pneumonia, and pulmonary edema, usually result in hypocapnia rather than hypercapnia [6]. In these cases, hypoxia stimulates ventilation; since carbon dioxide is much more diffusible (20 times) than oxygen, despite the gas exchange impairment, excretion of carbon dioxide is increased, and therefore pCO_2 levels fall. Other causes of respiratory alkalosis include bacterial toxins, Gram-negative septicemia, hepatic failure, and salicylate poisoning. Tables 6.1 and 6.2 show the important etiologies of acute and chronic respiratory acidosis and alkalosis, respectively.

6.2 Mechanisms in Respiratory Acidosis

Considering Eq. (4.2):

$$H_2O + CO_2 \rightleftharpoons H^+ + HCO_3^- \quad (4.2)$$

and Henderson-Hasselbalch equation for the above system (Eq. (3.5)):

$$pH = pK + \log \frac{\left[HCO_3^-\right]}{\alpha\, pCO_2} \quad (3.5)$$

any increase in arterial pCO_2, regardless of its cause, is followed by a proportionate increase in serum [H^+] and, thus, a decrease in blood *pH*. The resulting acidemia can be relieved only by a secondary increase in plasma $\left[HCO_3^-\right]$. In other words, the fraction $\left[HCO_3^-\right]/\left(\alpha\, pCO_2\right)$ decreases as the denominator (pCO_2) increases, and this causes a fall in *pH* (Henderson-Hasselbalch equation). The acidemia can be

Table 6.1 Common causes of acute respiratory acidosis and alkalosis

Acidosis	Alkalosis
Cardiac arrest	Anxiety, hysteria
Cardiogenic shock	Pulmonary emboli
Severe pulmonary edema	Mild pulmonary edema
Severe pneumonia	Mild pneumonia
Respiratory distress syndrome	$\dot{V}/\dot{Q}$ mismatch
Aspiration of foreign body	Congestive heart failure
Bronchospasm, laryngospasm	Hypotension
Pneumothorax, hemothorax	Decreased inspiratory pO_2
Flail chest	High altitude residence
Drug toxicity (e.g., curare, phenobarbital, succinylcholine, organophosphate, aminoglycosides [high dose])	Severe anemia
	Drug toxicity (e.g., salicylate, nicotine, dinitrophenol, methylxanthine derivatives [e.g., aminophylline])
Head injury	Head injury
Guillain Barré syndrome	Brain tumor or infection
Tetanus	Cerebrovascular accident
Botulism poisoning	Fever
Severe hypokalemia	Gram-negative septicemia
Severe hypophosphatemia	CO poisoning
General anesthesia	Mechanical overventilation
Mechanical underventilation	
Myasthenic crisis	

Table 6.2 Common causes of chronic respiratory acidosis and alkalosis

Acidosis	Alkalosis
COPD	Anxiety
Prolonged pneumonia	Hepatic failure with hepatic encephalopathy
Tracheal stenosis	Interstitial lung disease
Restrictive diseases of thorax	Interstitial fibrosis
Fibrothorax, hydrothorax	Severe anemia
Pleural effusion	Head injury
Scleroderma	Pregnancy
Interstitial fibrosis	Progesterone-producing tumor
Extreme obesity	Cyanotic heart disease
Ascites	
Kyphoscoliosis	
Muscular dystrophy	
Multiple sclerosis	
Amyotrophic lateral sclerosis	
Poliomyelitis	
Diaphragmatic paralysis	
Brain tumor or infection	

ameliorated by a proportionate rise in the numerator of the fraction $\left[HCO_3^-\right]/\left(\alpha\, pCO_2\right)$, that is an increase in $\left[HCO_3^-\right]$. The notable point with respect to bicarbonate is that the response develops in two steps: the first step or the *acute phase*, which is performed by cellular or tissue buffering capacity, and the second step which takes more time and depends on renal compensatory mechanisms [7]. The passage from acute to chronic stage may therefore be defined as the point at which the renal compensation for a primary respiratory acidosis becomes evident.

6.2.1 Acute Phase of Respiratory Acidosis

Hypercapnia immediately causes the reversible reaction:

$$H_2O + CO_2 \rightleftharpoons H^+ + HCO_3^- \tag{4.2}$$

proceeds to the right (Le Chatelier's principle), and as a consequence, plasma $\left[HCO_3^-\right]$ and [H^+] are increased. These surplus hydrogen ions are buffered by non-bicarbonate buffers, e.g., hemoglobin and intracellular proteins. Removal of H^+ ions causes the above reaction proceeds to the right more, thus the plasma $\left[HCO_3^-\right]$ will rise accordingly. However, the increment in plasma $\left[HCO_3^-\right]$ amounts to only 3–4 mEq/L, even with extreme hypercapnia (pCO_2 of 80–90 mm Hg). This small change in serum $\left[HCO_3^-\right]$ is sufficient to alleviate the severe acidemia that would otherwise ensue. If there is no further rise in arterial pCO_2, this adjustment is completed within 5–10 min and is followed by a stable period of a few hours, during which no further modifications in acid-base equilibrium take place. The net result is to increase plasma [H^+] and $\left[HCO_3^-\right]$ by about 0.75 nEq/L, and 0.1 mEq/L for each mm Hg increase in arterial pCO_2, respectively [8]:

$$\left.\begin{aligned} \Delta\left[HCO_3^-\right] &= 0.1\Delta pCO_2 \pm 2 \\ \Delta\left[H^+\right] &= 0.75\Delta pCO_2 \end{aligned}\right\} \tag{6.1}$$

6.2.2 Chronic Phase of Respiratory Acidosis

Conditions change when an elevation of arterial pCO_2 remains stable for several hours. The elevated pCO_2 diminishes the intracellular *pH* of the renal tubular cells, thus accelerating tubular acid secretion and generation of new bicarbonate. *As bicarbonate stores are augmented by this process, chloride stores are depleted*, as the majority of the excreted acid is in the form of ammonium chloride. Moreover, serum chloride concentration decreases due to chloride shift (Fig. 4.9) during the acute phase. After some degree of renal compensation, the system reaches a new equilibrium state in which, for a given elevation in arterial pCO_2, a new steady-state serum $\left[HCO_3^-\right]$ emerges. According to the clinical investigations (e.g., in patients with chronic obstructive lung disease), it is found that in chronic respiratory acidosis there is an association between the degree of hypercapnia and the elevated plasma $\left[HCO_3^-\right]$, after full physiologic compensation (Eq. (6.2)):

$$\left.\begin{aligned}\Delta\left[HCO_3^-\right] &= 0.4\Delta pCO_2 \pm 2\\ \Delta\left[H^+\right] &= 0.3\Delta pCO_2\end{aligned}\right\} \tag{6.2}$$

Thus, although normal *pH* is not re-established, in chronic hypercapnia, the blood *pH* is preserved better than that in acute conditions.

6.3 Clinical Manifestations of Respiratory Acidosis

The clinical symptoms of respiratory acidosis vary greatly, depending on the rapidity with which the hypercapnia ensues. Different neurological abnormalities can be produced by severe acute respiratory acidosis. The first symptoms include headache, blurred vision, restlessness, and marked anxiety, which can progress to tremor, asterixis, delirium, somnolence, confusion, stupor, and even coma. The cerebrospinal fluid (CSF) pressure is often raised and papilledema may be present. The latter effects may be in part due to the increased cerebral blood flow, which is caused by hypercapnia. In general, chronic respiratory acidosis is better tolerated than the acute form with the same degree of elevation of pCO_2.

A decline in alveolar ventilation is always accompanied by a certain degree of hypoxia in those breathing room air; the hypoxia may also contribute to symptomatology. In addition, acidemia may reduce the myocardial contractility and performance. Various cardiac arrhythmias and peripheral vasodilation may also occur, which result in severe hypotension if the systemic *pH* drops to less than 7.1. Hypercapnia reduces peripheral vascular resistance by causing vasodilation in most arterial beds. However, it may also cause venoconstriction and a resulting redistribution of blood from the periphery to the pulmonary circulation. Hypercapnia can produce some catecholamine release, however, in itself, it lessens cardiovascular response to a given level of catecholamines. Normally, during moderately severe acute respiratory acidosis, the cardiac output and systemic blood pressure are well preserved. Cardiovascular function may nonetheless be disturbed with extreme acidemia (e.g., due to the superimposed lactate acidosis), or in case of a primary circulatory problem.

6.4 Diagnosis of Respiratory Acidosis

The physical findings of bradypnea, depressed respiratory effort, and past history of chronic lung disease can indicate the existence of a respiratory acidosis. Diagnosis should not be difficult considering laboratory data—coexistence of acidemia ($pH < 7.35$) and hypercapnia ($p_aCO_2 > 45$ mm Hg) associated with a proportionate hyperbicarbia (Eqs. (6.1) and (6.2)) is diagnostic for respiratory acidosis. To find the underlying disorder, one must pay attention to the history of the patient. Do not forget that *there is no substitute for an accurate and comprehensive history.*

Example A previously healthy 4-year-old boy is brought to the emergency room with a history of sudden onset of vomiting and severe cough. At the time, he developed the symptoms when he was playing; the parents reported no preceding events. On arrival, the examining doctor observed that the patient was severely dyspneic, confused, and mildly cyanotic.

Arterial blood gas analysis reveals a $pCO_2 = 60$ mm Hg, $\left[HCO_3^-\right] = 27$ mEq/L, $pH = 7.275$, and a BE of −0.48 mEq/L. What is the diagnosis?

Solution: A low pH (7.275) with a high pCO_2 (60 mm Hg) indicates a respiratory acidosis. The BE is within normal range (Table 6.1), and the raise in serum $\left[HCO_3^-\right]$ (3 mEq/L = 27–24) is compatible with an acute process (Eq. (6.1)):

$$\begin{aligned}\Delta\left[HCO_3^-\right] &= 0.1\Delta pCO_2 \pm 2\\ &= 0.1\times(60-40)\pm 2\\ &= 0.1\times 20\pm 2\\ &= 2\pm 2\,\text{mEq}/\text{L}\end{aligned}$$

This clinical picture directs the physician to the cause of the disturbance—acute airway obstruction. Bronchoscopy revealed a marble in the patient's trachea (perhaps the one he was playing with). Normal acid-base status was restored, as soon as the obstruction was removed.

Example A 60-year-old woman, a known case of chronic obstructive pulmonary disease (COPD), was hospitalized with the diagnosis of *cor-pulmonale*. On admission, the arterial blood gas analysis showed the following values:

$pCO_2 = 60$ mm Hg, $\left[HCO_3^-\right] = 31$ mEq/L, $pH = 7.335$, BE = 4.03 mEq/L.

What is the acid-base status?

Solution: Considering the blood pH (7.335), the patient has acidemia ($pH < 7.35$). Regarding blood pCO_2 (60 mm Hg), and $\left[HCO_3^-\right]$ (31 mEq/L), the underlying cause should be a respiratory problem. The measured $\Delta\left[HCO_3^-\right]$ (7 mEq/L = 31–24) is consistent with a chronic respiratory acidosis (Eq. (6.2)):

$$\begin{aligned}\Delta\left[HCO_3^-\right] &= 0.4\Delta pCO_2 \pm 2\\ &= 0.4\times(60-40)\pm 2\\ &= 0.4\times 20\pm 2\\ &= 8\pm 2\,\text{mEq}/\text{L}\end{aligned}$$

The positive BE (4.03 > 2) is also in favor of our diagnosis (either metabolic alkalosis or compensated respiratory acidosis). This acid-base condition is reasonably expected if we look precisely at the patient's history (COPD).

As it can be clearly seen, in spite of the same change in arterial pCO_2 (20 mm Hg), the blood *pH* of the patient in this example was better preserved than that of the patient in the previous example (7.335 vs. 7.275). Obviously, this difference is because of the *renal compensation for respiratory acidosis*, which was explained earlier.

6.5 Treatment of Respiratory Acidosis

Management of acute respiratory acidosis must be focused on eliminating the underlying cause. The *immediate priority is to restore a satisfactory ventilation*, in order to prevent severe hypoxia [8].

Because even with severe chronic hypercapnia, there is only a moderate decrease in blood *pH*, no treatment is usually necessary for those with well-compensated pure chronic respiratory acidosis. The therapy should be directed at *removing the underlying etiology*, commonly a chronic lung disease. Ventilation should be improved by any possible means, be it through bronchodilators use, administration of antibiotics for lung infection, chest physiotherapy and postural drainage, or giving diuretics for congestive heart failure. Acute exacerbation of obstructive lung disease may need periods of assisted ventilation.

6.6 Mechanisms in Respiratory Alkalosis

In respiratory alkalosis, similar changes happen, but in an opposite direction. Let us look again at Eq. (4.2):

$$H_2O + CO_2 \rightleftharpoons H^+ + HCO_3^- \tag{4.2}$$

As arterial pCO_2 falls (hypocapnia), as a result of alveolar hyperventilation, the foregoing reaction proceeds to the left and a consequent drop in serum $[H^+]$, and $\left[HCO_3^-\right]$ ensues. Stated differently, regarding the Henderson-Hasselbalch equation (Eq. (3.5)):

$$pH = pK + \log\frac{\left[HCO_3^-\right]}{\alpha\, pCO_2} \tag{3.5}$$

hypocapnia (a fall in arterial pCO_2) decreases the denominator of the fraction $\left[HCO_3^-\right]/\left(\alpha\, pCO_2\right)$, and produces an increase in blood *pH* (alkalemia). The resulting alkalemia can be alleviated only by a secondary decrease in plasma $\left[HCO_3^-\right]$. As in respiratory acidosis, here again the response occurs in two phases.

6.6.1 Acute Phase of Respiratory Alkalosis

In the acute phase, non-bicarbonate buffers (e.g., hemoglobin and proteins) play the major role. These act within minutes and cause a decrease in plasma $\left[HCO_3^-\right]$ which amounts to 3–4 mEq/L as the arterial pCO_2 falls to 20–25 mm Hg. Note that the initial decrement in bicarbonate level depicts a larger change in response to the alteration in arterial pCO_2 than the initial increment in the acute hypercapnia, which is limited to 3–4 mEq/L even when hypercapnia is severe. Generally, in the acute phase of respiratory alkalosis, the plasma bicarbonate concentration drops by 2 mEq/L for each 10 mm Hg decrease in arterial pCO_2. This correction is fulfilled within 5–10 min and is followed by a stable period of a few hours [7]. The net result is to decrease plasma hydrogen ion concentration by about 0.75 nEq/L for each mm Hg fall in arterial pCO_2 (as in acute respiratory acidosis) (Eq. (6.3)):

$$\left.\begin{aligned}\Delta\left[HCO_3^-\right] &= 0.2\Delta pCO_2 \pm 2\\ \Delta\left[H^+\right] &= 0.75\Delta pCO_2\end{aligned}\right\} \tag{6.3}$$

6.6.2 Chronic Phase of Respiratory Alkalosis

As in respiratory acidosis, here again the kidneys play an important role in compensation of alkalosis. The reduced arterial pCO_2 decreases the $[H^+]$ in the renal tubular cells and, as a consequence, the sodium-hydrogen exchange (Figs. 4.11 and 4.12) is dampened. Net acid excretion and rate of bicarbonate reabsorption are decreased and, as a result, there is an additional drop in plasma $\left[HCO_3^-\right]$. These adjustments are completed within 2–4 days. Thereafter, the system reaches a new equilibrium state in which the plasma $\left[HCO_3^-\right]$ and $[H^+]$ are decreased by about 5 mEq/L, and 3 nEq/L for each 10 mm Hg fall in arterial pCO_2, respectively:

$$\left.\begin{aligned}\Delta\left[HCO_3^-\right] &= 0.5\Delta pCO_2 \pm 2\\ \Delta\left[H^+\right] &= 0.3\Delta pCO_2\end{aligned}\right\} \tag{6.4}$$

Note that the change in $[H^+]$ is similar to what it was in chronic respiratory acidosis (Eq. (6.2)).

6.7 Clinical Manifestations of Respiratory Alkalosis

The symptoms of respiratory alkalosis are related to increased irritability of the central and peripheral nervous system. The typical manifestation of acute respiratory alkalosis is numbness and tingling of the lips and extremities [8]. Hyperventilation causes hypocapnia which leads to increased resistance in cerebral circulation; cerebral blood flow reduces as much as 35%–40%, if arterial pCO_2 falls by 20 mm Hg. Hence, the patient feels light-headed and dizzy. Furthermore, the patient may suffer from muscle spasms due to decreased fraction of ionized calcium in the blood. Finally, in case of severe alkalemia, syncope, seizure, and an altered level of consciousness may arise. A variety of cardiac arrhythmias may occur, particularly in seriously ill patients. These abnormalities are believed to be related to the ability of alkalosis to impair cerebral function and to increase membrane excitability.

Patients with psychogenic hyperventilation often complain of symptoms which are actually not related to alkalemia. For example, they may complain of headache, shortness of breath, chest pain or tightness, and other somatic symptoms, which may be emotional in origin.

The above symptoms predominantly develop in acute respiratory alkalosis when the arterial pCO_2 drops below 25–30 mm Hg. They are much less likely to be seen in chronic states. An additional finding in many patients with severe respiratory alkalosis, which is caused from the rapid shift of extracellular phosphate into the cells, is a decline in plasma phosphate concentration to as low as 0.5–1.5 mg/dL (reference range: 2.5–4.5 mg/dL). This phenomenon needs no special treatment, but the physician should be aware of its presence, since further evaluation for the other causes of hypophosphatemia is no longer indicated.

6.8 Diagnosis of Respiratory Alkalosis

The physical finding of tachypnea may be a clue for the presence of a respiratory alkalosis. Diagnosis should not be difficult regarding laboratory findings; an alkaline blood ($pH > 7.45$) associated with hypocapnia ($pCO_2 < 35$ mm Hg) and a proportionate hypobicarbia (Eqs. (6.3) and (6.4)) confirm the existence of a respiratory alkalosis. Nevertheless, do not forget that a *complete history-taking and physical examination are essential for the correct interpretation of acid-base status.*

Example An 18-year-old woman complained of severe dyspnea after learning of the death of her mother. Examination disclosed a respiratory rate of 40/min, carpopedal spasm, and cold moist skin. Arterial blood gas analysis was reported as:

$pCO_2 = 25$ mm Hg, $\left[HCO_3^-\right] = 20.2$ mEq/L, $pH = 7.529$, BE = 0.19 mEq/L. What is your diagnosis?

Solution: The high pH (7.529), with the low pCO_2 (25 mm Hg) and $\left[HCO_3^-\right]$ (20.2 mEq/L), is consistent with an acute respiratory alkalosis (due to hyperventilation). Using Eq. (6.3), it can be seen that the change in $\left[HCO_3^-\right]$ (3.8 mEq/L = 24–20.2) is also consistent with an acute process:

$$\begin{aligned} \Delta\left[HCO_3^-\right] &= 0.2\Delta pCO_2 \pm 2 \\ &= 0.2 \times (40 - 25) \pm 2 \\ &= 0.2 \times 15 \pm 2 \\ &= 3 \pm 2\,\text{mEq/L} \end{aligned}$$

The presence of hyperventilation and tachypnea with a normal BE (0.19 < 2) are all in favor of an acute respiratory alkalosis. The treatment for the patient consists of mild sedation and breathing into and out of a paper bag (to increase inspired CO_2 partial pressure).

Example The arterial blood gas analysis of a comatose patient admitted to the neurosurgical ICU reveals the following values:

$pCO_2 = 25$ mm Hg, $\left[HCO_3^-\right] = 17$ mEq/L, $pH = 7.454$, BE = −4.82 mEq/L. What is the acid-base-status?

Solution: The high *pH* (7.454) indicates alkalemia. Regarding low pCO_2 (25 mm Hg) and $\left[HCO_3^-\right]$ (17 mEq/L) and proportionate decrease in $\left[HCO_3^-\right]$:

$$\begin{aligned}\Delta\left[HCO_3^-\right] &= 0.5\Delta pCO_2 \pm 2\\ &= 0.5\times(40-25)\pm 2\\ &= 0.5\times 15\pm 2\\ &= 7.5\pm 2\,\text{mEq / L}\end{aligned}$$

The diagnosis is clear—chronic respiratory alkalosis. Again, as it can be seen, in chronic states blood *pH* is preserved better than that in the acute phase.

6.9 Treatment of Respiratory Alkalosis

In general, treatment of the alkalemia is unnecessary; instead, *efforts should be made to remove the underlying cause* [8]. In the severely symptomatic patient with acute respiratory alkalosis, his breathing into a paper bag elevates the pCO_2 of the inspired air; this may therefore partially correct the existing hypocapnia and alleviate the symptoms.

Example A 56-year-old man is noted to be tachypneic and confused 2 days after suffering multiple injuries in a car accident. Chest roentgenogram is unremarkable. His arterial blood gas values are as follows:

$pCO_2 = 30$ mm Hg, $\left[HCO_3^-\right] = 21$ mEq/L, $pH = 7.467$, BE = −0.48 mEq/L. What is the most likely problem with this patient?

Solution: The alkalemia concomitant with hypocapnia and a proportionate drop in serum $\left[HCO_3^-\right]$, all confirm an acute respiratory alkalosis. Normal value of BE is also compatible with the condition. Normal chest X-ray and the clinical *triad of dyspnea, confusion, and petechia* in a person who has had recent long-bone fracture corroborates the diagnosis of *fat embolism syndrome*. The time course of events is also consistent with our diagnosis.

Example A previously healthy 21-year-old lady was admitted to the hospital in a coma. She was diagnosed with major depressive disorder previously and drug overdose was thus suspected. The respiratory rate was 10/min and she was cyanotic. Arterial blood gas analysis was reported as follows:

$pCO_2 = 92$ mm Hg, $\left[HCO_3^-\right] = 30$ mEq/L, $pH = 7.135$, BE = −0.43 mEq/L. What is the most appropriate treatment for the woman described above?

Solution: The acidemia associated with the very high pCO_2 and the harmonious change in blood $\left[HCO_3^-\right]$ reveals an acute respiratory acidosis. The normal BE also agrees with this situation. As acidosis must be rapidly reversed by increased ventilation, endotracheal intubation should be performed; mechanical ventilation to a sufficient amount should be started to return arterial *pH* to a physiologic range.

6.10 Things to Remember

Any factor that decreases pulmonary ventilation causes a respiratory acidosis. On the contrary, excessive pulmonary ventilation leads to respiratory alkalosis (Tables 6.1 and 6.2).

The compensation for respiratory acid-base derangements is started early, primarily by non-bicarbonate buffers (acute phase), and then is followed by renal compensation (chronic phase), which by adjusting the rate of reabsorption and synthesis of bicarbonate controls the blood $\left[HCO_3^-\right]$ and *pH*.

Considering blood *pH*, $\left[HCO_3^-\right]$, pCO_2, the history and physical examination, the diagnosis is easy. In the acute phase, the BE usually shows little or no change at all, but in chronic respiratory acidosis and alkalosis it is positive and negative, respectively (Table 6.3).

In almost all cases, the treatment should be focused on eliminating the underlying cause.

Table 6.3 Changes in blood chemistry in respiratory acid-base disorders

Condition	*pH*	pCO_2	$\left[HCO_3^-\right]$	BE
Acute R. Ac.	↓↓	↑	$\uparrow: \Delta\left[HCO_3^-\right] = 0.1\Delta pCO_2 \pm 2$	Nl.
Chronic R. Ac.	↓	↑	$\uparrow: \Delta\left[HCO_3^-\right] = 0.4\Delta pCO_2 \pm 2$	>2
Acute R. Al.	↑↑	↓	$\downarrow: \Delta\left[HCO_3^-\right] = 0.2\Delta pCO_2 \pm 2$	Nl.
Chronic R. Al.	↑	↓	$\downarrow: \Delta\left[HCO_3^-\right] = 0.5\Delta pCO_2 \pm 2$	<−2

R. Ac. Respiratory acidosis, R. Al. Respiratory alkalosis, Nl. Normal

References

1. Epstein SK, Singh N. Respiratory acidosis. Respir Care. 2001;46(4):366–83.
2. Foster GT, Vaziri ND, Sassoon CS. Respiratory alkalosis. Respir Care. 2001;46(4):384–91.
3. Patel S, Sharma S. Respiratory acidosis. Treasure Island, FL: StatPearls; 2020.
4. Ghimire P, Kaul P. Pickwickian Syndrome. Treasure Island, FL: StatPearls; 2020.
5. Brinkman JE, Sharma S. Respiratory Alkalosis. Treasure Island, FL: StatPearls; 2020.
6. West JB. Respiratory physiology. 9th ed. Philadelphia: Lippincott Williams and Wilkins; 2012.
7. Kassirer JP, Madias NE. Respiratory acid-base disorders. Hosp Pract. 1980;15(12):57–9., 65-71. https://doi.org/10.1080/21548331.1980.11946696.
8. Narins RG, Gardner LB. Simple acid-base disturbances. Med Clin North Am. 1981;65(2):321–46. https://doi.org/10.1016/s0025-7125(16)31527-9.

Metabolic Acidosis and Alkalosis

7

Definition In the previous chapter, it was seen that in respiratory acid-base disturbances, the primary cause is a change in pCO_2. Now, in this chapter, the consequences of a primary alteration in serum bicarbonate level, i.e., metabolic (non-respiratory) acid-base imbalances will be explained.

Reconsidering the following equation, and Le Chatelier's principle:

$$H_2O + CO_2 \rightleftharpoons H_2CO_3 \rightleftharpoons H^+ + HCO_3^-$$

any decrease in plasma $\left[HCO_3^-\right]$ proceeds the above equation to the right and, ultimately, causes an increase in serum $[H^+]$. These surplus hydrogen ions result in an acidosis (by definition), and as this arises following a non-respiratory abnormality, the condition is known as *metabolic* (non-respiratory) acidosis [1].

On the contrary, increased plasma $\left[HCO_3^-\right]$ reverts the above process. The reaction shifts to the left; the excess $\left[HCO_3^-\right]$ ions combine with H^+ ions to form carbonic acid (H_2CO_3) which dissociates to CO_2 and water. The primary increased body bicarbonate store is defined as alkalosis, and as this is not due to a respiratory problem (i.e., hyperventilation or tachypnea), the condition is termed metabolic (non-respiratory) alkalosis. The variation in serum $[H^+]$ in metabolic acidosis or alkalosis produces acidemia (a decrease in blood *pH*) or alkalemia (an increase in blood *pH*), respectively.

7.1 Pathogenesis and Compensatory Mechanisms

7.1.1 Metabolic Acidosis

In a normal adult, because of the cellular metabolism, about 50–100 mEq acid (1–1.5 mEq/kg/day) in the form of sulfuric acid (H_2SO_4), phosphoric acid (H_3PO_4), and other various organic acids are formed daily. These non-volatile (non-bicarbonic

F. Habibzadeh et al., *Pathophysiologic Basis of Acid-Base Disorders*,
https://doi.org/10.1007/978-981-16-0526-0_7

or fixed) acids are usually excreted by the kidney, and their accumulation results in acidemia (increased [H^+]). Hydrogen ion, due to its electrical charge, cannot cross the blood-brain barrier (BBB) readily, but it causes the reversible reaction

$$H_2O + CO_2 \rightleftharpoons H^+ + HCO_3^- \quad (4.2)$$

proceeds to the left. Thus, the plasma CO_2 tension is increased (do not forget that at the first stage, the increase in [H^+] occurs only in plasma, a phenomenon the cerebrospinal fluid (CSF) is unaware of). The produced CO_2 easily crosses BBB and elevates the CSF CO_2 partial pressure. The increased CSF pCO_2 causes the above reaction in the CSF to proceed to the right (meanwhile, the reaction in the plasma carries on from right to left). CO_2 reacts with water to form H^+ again. The resultant acid CSF bathes the H^+-sensitive medullary respiratory center and causes hyperventilation, which in turn decreases the plasma pCO_2. Thereby, the above reaction in plasma shifts to the left, excess H^+ is removed, plasma $\left[HCO_3^-\right]$ is reduced, and blood *pH* returns toward, but not to, a normal value. This is the *respiratory compensation for metabolic acidosis.*

The same events also occur in the kidney and decrease the intracellular *pH* of the tubular cell. As was explained earlier, this in turn causes the kidney to excrete more acid (acid urine), and generate new bicarbonate. Therefore, the body compensation for a metabolic acidosis is a pulmonary-renal mechanism and, in general, includes:

1. an immediate response by blood buffers (within minutes),
2. a quick response by respiratory hyperventilation (within hours), and
3. a slow-acting renal compensation (within days).

7.1.2 Metabolic Alkalosis

In contrary to what was seen in metabolic acidosis, decreased plasma [H^+] causes the reaction

$$H_2O + CO_2 \rightleftharpoons H^+ + HCO_3^- \quad (4.2)$$

proceeds to the right (Le Chatelier's principle), and as a consequence, the plasma pCO_2 falls. Here again H^+, because of its electrical charge, cannot cross BBB instantly, but CSF CO_2, which is in equilibrium with plasma CO_2, penetrates through BBB to the plasma under its concentration (partial pressure) gradient. The CSF pCO_2 declines and the above reaction (Eq. (4.2)) shifts to the left, which results in an alkaline CSF. This alkaline CSF depresses the medullary respiratory centers and causes hypoventilation. These cause CO_2 accumulation, progression of Eq. (4.2) to the right, and increase the plasma [H^+] toward, but not to, normal. This is the *respiratory compensation for a metabolic alkalosis*. However, this hypoventilatory response is *restricted by hypoxemia* so that arterial pCO_2 seldom rises above 55 mm Hg—values above this level are usually associated with an arterial pO_2 below 65 mm Hg. Nevertheless, considerable inter-individual variability in the upper limit of the arterial pCO_2 is well appreciated and is affected by arterial pO_2 and $[K^+]$, among other things.

Hypokalemia restricts the level of respiratory compensation with two possible mechanisms: first, there may have been redistribution of H^+ ions into cells of the respiratory center as a consequence of hypokalemia; and second, potassium depletion per se may have changed the respiratory neural activity.

Although the same events occur in the intracellular space of the renal tubular cells, the kidney may react in another way. Effective arterial blood volume and organ perfusion is carefully secured by the kidneys. The perception of hypovolemia results in intense renal water and salt retention. Sodium is reabsorbed regardless of whether its accompanying anion is Cl^- or $\left[HCO_3^-\right]$, even in the presence of a high serum $\left[HCO_3^-\right]$. Thus, hypovolemia, which is one of the causes of metabolic alkalosis, stimulates so potently sodium reabsorption that the kidneys sacrifice body fluid tonicity and acid-base balance, to preserve volume. This is why the hypercarbonatemic hypovolemic states (e.g., vomiting and over-diuresis) are usually associated with a urine poor in Na^+ and $\left[HCO_3^-\right]$, indicating avid renal $NaHCO_3$ reabsorption. Re-expansion of extracellular fluid removes the kidney from the constrains of hypovolemia, allowing the filtered $\left[HCO_3^-\right]$ to be excreted into the urine and dampens the mechanism involving the generation of new bicarbonate. Therefore, the compensatory mechanism for metabolic alkalosis is also a pulmonary-renal one.

As in respiratory acid-base disorders, employing the Henderson-Hasselbalch equation (Eq. (3.5)), the process involving metabolic acid-base disturbances can also be explained in another way. The discussion is left as an exercise for the reader.

7.2 Causes of Metabolic Acidosis

There is a balance between production, buffering, and excretion of acids. Any disturbance in this physiologic system would result in accumulation of fixed acid and hypobicarbonatemia, the hallmarks of metabolic acidosis. Metabolic acidosis may arise due to:

1. over-production of non-volatile (non-bicarbonic or fixed) acid,
2. loss of extracellular bicarbonate, and
3. decreased renal acid excretion.

7.2.1 Over-Production of Fixed Acid

Fat, carbohydrate, and sulfur-containing amino acids are metabolized to form fixed acids such as sulfuric or phosphoric acids. The produced acid is then buffered by bicarbonate and eventually either excreted from the kidney or expelled from the lung in the form of CO_2. Usually, this system is in an equilibrium state, and the rate of acid production is just equal to its removal. The acid load may be increased either by acid over-production (e.g., ketoacidosis, lactic acidosis), or because of an external source (e.g., toxicity with salicylate, ethylene glycol, paraldehyde). In such cases, more bicarbonate is needed to buffer the overloaded acid, and subsequently, the bicarbonate store will be diminished and a metabolic acidosis may ensue.

7.2.2 Loss of Buffer Stores (Bicarbonate Wasting)

Alkali may be lost from the kidney (e.g., *proximal renal tubular acidosis* (RTA) [2]) or from the gastrointestinal tract (e.g., diarrhea).

7.2.3 Decreased Normal Renal Acid Excretion

Conditions with associated renal impairment to excrete acid may result in acid retention and, therefore, metabolic acidosis [3, 4]. Examples of such conditions are renal failure and distal renal tubular acidosis (type I RTA) [2]. Renal failure causes decreased glomerular filtration; thus, the produced organic acids are not removed from the body and, as a consequence, a metabolic acidosis ensues. However, in distal RTA, the pathophysiology is different; the mechanism involving tubular acid secretion does not work properly, and it is the accumulation of these H^+ ions which results in a metabolic acidosis [2].

By a careful history-taking, physical examination, and a few simple laboratory tests, one can simply determine the nature of the existing metabolic acidosis. The change in *AG* can be an important clue in approaching the metabolic acidosis. Clinically, metabolic acidosis can be classified into: (1) *normal-AG (hyperchloremic)* [5], and (2) *high-AG acidosis* [6] (Table 7.1). In normal-*AG* acidosis, an equal amount of plasma bicarbonate is replaced by an equal amount of chloride, that is, the decrease in serum $\left[HCO_3^-\right]$ is just equal to the increase in serum $[Cl^-]$. Thereby, the *AG* remains unchanged.

Table 7.1 Classification, causes, and mechanisms of metabolic acidosis

Classification	Mechanism
Normal-AG (hyperchloremic) acidosis	
I. Hypokalemic acidosis	
A. RTA	
1. Proximal RTA (type II)	Defect in bicarbonate reabsorption in proximal tubule
2. Distal RTA (type I)	Impaired distal tubule acidification
B. GI disturbances	
1. Diarrhea	Loss of bicarbonate in stool and increased acid production by bacteria in stool
2. Biliary or pancreatic fistula	Loss of bicarbonate into bile or pancreatic secretion

Table 7.1 (continued)

Classification	Mechanism
C. Drugs and toxins	
1. Carbonic anhydrase inhibitors (e.g., acetazolamide)	Impaired proximal tubule acid excretion
2. Amphotericin B	Induced RTA
3. Toluene toxicity	Induced RTA and accumulation of organic acids
D. Ureteral diversion	
1. Ureterosigmoidostomy	Increased bicarbonate loss into the feces
2. Ileal bladder	Increased ammonia reabsorption which liberates H^+
3. Ileal ureter	Infection, reflux, and its secondary changes such as loss of renal mass
II. Normokalemic or hyperkalemic acidosis	
A. Hyper-alimentation	Cationic amino acids (lysine, arginine, histidine), whose anion (Cl^-) is metabolized and produces neutral substances and HCl
B. Early renal failure and hydronephrosis	Volume expansion produces dilution of bicarbonate with a constant pCO_2. Defect in H^+ excretion accompanying normal GFR
C. Exogenous acid	Addition of HCl, NH_4Cl, Arg-HCl, Lys-HCl, $CaCl_2$, and cholestyramine
D. Hypoaldosteronism 1. Primary adrenal disorder 2. Low renin secretion 3. Renal tubular resistance to aldosterone	Reduced net renal acid excretion predominantly by decreased ammonia excretion.
E. Drugs (e.g., spironolactone)	Excess serum K^+ (due to blockade of aldosterone) and reduced urinary K^+ excretion reduce renal ammonia excretion which results in acidosis.
F. Post-hypocapnic acidosis	Hypocapnia stimulates renal acid retention and bicarbonaturia (renal compensation for respiratory alkalosis). During treatment of respiratory alkalosis the rise in pCO_2 is faster than that for plasma $\left[HCO_3^-\right]$, which results in a transient metabolic acidosis.
G. Sulfur toxicity	Sulfur-containing amino acids (e.g., methionine, cystine, and cysteine) are metabolized to sulfuric acid. Sodium sulfate is filtered by kidney and is poorly reabsorbed. The H^+ accumulates and the anion is replaced by Cl^-, thus, a normal-*AG* acidosis occurs.
High-AG acidosis	
A. Renal failure	Impaired synthesis or reabsorption of bicarbonate in the kidney
B. Ketoacidosis	Accumulation of acetoacetic and β-hydroxybutyric acid
C. Lactic acidosis	Accumulation of lactic acid
D. Toxins	
1. Methanol	Accumulation of end-products of methanol (e.g., formaldehyde and formic acid)
2. Ethylene glycol	Accumulation of end-products of ethylene glycol (e.g., oxalic acid and hippuric acid)
3. Salicylate intoxication	Probable accumulation of lactic acid and ketoacids

7.3 Causes of Metabolic Alkalosis

Over-production of bicarbonate in the kidney, secondary to excess of mineralocorticoid hormones, diuretic therapy, or volume contraction may increase plasma $\left[HCO_3^-\right]$. In volume contraction, serum $\left[HCO_3^-\right]$ is increased because of:

1. decreased volume with a constant bicarbonate content causes the plasma $\left[HCO_3^-\right]$ to be raised
2. volume contraction stimulates proximal tubular Na^+ reabsorption in exchange for H^+ and K^+. For each milliequivalent of H^+ excreted into the urine, one milliequivalent of $\left[HCO_3^-\right]$ is added to the blood. Loss of H^+ and K^+ in the urine will ultimately cause a hypokalemic metabolic alkalosis [7].

Loss of gastric acid, for example, as a result of prolonged nasogastric suction or vomiting, also produces a metabolic alkalosis. The stomach (like the kidneys) hydrates CO_2 to form H_2CO_3, which ionizes to H^+ and $\left[HCO_3^-\right]$. The hydrogen ion then secrets to the gastric fluid (or urine in the case of the kidneys). Meanwhile, the bicarbonate ion is added to the blood and results in a transient metabolic alkalosis. The entrance of acid gastric content into the duodenum stimulates the secretion of alkaline pancreatic juice (rich in $\left[HCO_3^-\right]$) which otherwise may cause a metabolic alkalosis. This process removes the surplus bicarbonate ions from the blood and guards the acid-base balance [8].

Exogenous administration of alkali, such as bicarbonate therapy, or massive blood transfusion, may produce metabolic alkalosis. Each unit of whole blood or packed red cell contains 17 or 5 mEq of citrate, respectively. Consequently, massive blood transfusion causes a transient metabolic acidosis (because of free citric acid in the transfused blood), followed by a metabolic alkalosis (due to *conversion of citrate to bicarbonate in liver*). Patients with a normal kidney function can excrete this alkali load easily and develop no problems at all. Etiologic factors and mechanisms of metabolic alkalosis are shown in Table 7.2.

7.4 Systemic Manifestations of Metabolic Acidosis

The symptoms of metabolic acidosis are nonspecific. Patients with metabolic acidosis due to hypobicarbonatemia demonstrate tachypnea and hyperpnea, *Kussmaul's* or labored respiration, the latter of which is the most prominent physical finding, especially in acute (uncompensated) metabolic acidosis [1, 9]. The patient complains of fatigue, weakness, malaise (especially in chronic (compensated) metabolic acidosis), nausea, vomiting, and abdominal pain. In severe conditions, an altered level of consciousness, stupor, and even coma may occur.

Table 7.2 Causes and mechanisms of metabolic alkalosis

Condition	Mechanism of generation	Mechanism of maintenance
Loss of H^+		
A. *Extrarenal loss*		
1. GI tract (e.g., vomiting, gastric drainage, nasogastric suction, anti-acid therapy, congenital chloride loosing diarrhea	Loss of acid	Hypovolemia
2. Shift into cell (e.g., sustained hypokalemia)	Shift of H^+ into cell in exchange for K^+	
B. *Renal loss*		
1. Excess mineralocorticoids (e.g., primary aldosteronism, Cushing syndrome, Bartter's syndrome)	Increases renal H^+ secretion through its effect on Na^+ transport	Aldosterone excess, induced hypokalemia, and hypovolemia
2. Diuretic therapy (e.g., furosemide, ethacrynic acid, thiazide)	Reduces the extracellular fluid volume without any change in total body bicarbonate	Volume contraction and hypokalemia
3. Excretion of large amount of non-absorbable anions (e.g., SO_4^{2-}, HPO_4^{2-} in a Na^+-depleted patient; penicillin; carbenicillin)	K^+ and H^+ are excreted into tubular lumen in order to neutralize the electronegativity of these poorly reabsorbable anions.	Continued loss of K^+ and H^+
4. Severe hypokalemia	Hypokalemia enhances renal ammonia production and chlordiuresis.	Renal ammonia production and chlordiuresis
5. Post-hypercapnic alkalosis	The renal compensation for respiratory acidosis causes accumulation of $\left[HCO_3^-\right]$. Restoring normal ventilation in such conditions corrects arterial pCO_2, but leaves serum $\left[HCO_3^-\right]$ already high, thus, precipitating a metabolic alkalosis.	
Extracellular volume loss (e.g., GI tract [villous adenoma], skin [cystic fibrosis], kidney [heavy diuresis])	Volume contraction	Hypovolemia
Net gain of exogenous base (e.g., oral or parenteral bicarbonate administration, metabolic conversion of lactate and acetate to bicarbonate, and milk alkali syndrome)	Bicarbonate load produces volume contraction, K^+ depletion, and aldosterone excess. It also causes mobilization of H^+ in exchange for K^+ into cell	

7.5 Systemic Manifestations of Metabolic Alkalosis

The most common signs and symptoms of metabolic alkalosis are CNS manifestations including confusion, obtundation, delirium, and decreased seizure threshold. Other important clinical findings are positive *Chvostek's* and *Trousseau's* signs, increased muscular excitability, cardiac arrhythmia, and hypotension [10].

7.6 Diagnosis of Metabolic Acidosis

The studies of Albert, Dell, and Winter revealed that at the steady state, the arterial pCO_2 and plasma $\left[HCO_3^-\right]$ in a compensated metabolic acidosis are strongly correlated. This correlation can be expressed as the following equation (*Winter's* formula):

$$pCO_2 = 1.5\left[HCO_3^-\right] + 8 \pm 2 \tag{7.1}$$

Also, in an uncomplicated metabolic acidosis, the respiratory compensation causes the pCO_2 to decline by 1.1–1.4 mm Hg for each mEq/L decrease in serum $\left[HCO_3^-\right]$. If the measured pCO_2 is significantly higher than the predicted value from the formula, a complicating respiratory acidosis should also be considered. On the other hand, a measured pCO_2 lower than that predicted by the formula, notifies that the hyperventilatory response is out of proportion to the acidosis, and indicates the coexistence of a respiratory alkalosis.

As a rough estimate, the change in blood *pH* in a compensated metabolic acidosis can be nicely expressed as the equation:

$$pCO_2 \approx \left[HCO_3^-\right] + 15 \approx 2\,\text{digits after decimal point of blood}\ p\text{H} \tag{7.2}$$

As mentioned earlier, in acidosis an immediate response occurs by buffers and a new steady state is achieved within 12–36 h. Before reaching this equilibrium state, when the plasma bicarbonate concentration is low, and the pCO_2 is still falling (uncompensated metabolic acidosis), Winter's formula gives a false impression that the pCO_2 is inappropriately high for the measured serum $\left[HCO_3^-\right]$.

As was explained before, a negative base excess (base deficit) reveals an excess of non-volatile (non-bicarbonic, fixed) acid or deficiency of bicarbonate. Such conditions occur either in metabolic acidosis or compensated respiratory alkalosis. In these cases, considering the blood *pH*, acidemia reflects a metabolic acidosis, whereas alkalemia shows a compensated respiratory alkalosis.

Example A 26-year-old man, injured in a car accident, sustained a large hepatic laceration which was repaired at laparotomy. During the procedure, the systolic blood pressure intermittently dropped to 50 mm Hg and two units of blood were transfused to preserve an adequate pressure. Blood gas analysis, after stabilization post-operatively, was reported as follows:

$pCO_2 = 25$ mm Hg, $\left[HCO_3^-\right] = 12$ mEq/L, $pH = 7.303$, BE = −12.58 mEq/L.

Serum chemistry revealed:
$[Na^+] = 140$ mEq/L, $[K^+] = 4.1$ mEq/L, $[Cl^-] = 104$ mEq/L.
What is your diagnosis?

Solution: The *pH* is less than 7.35 (acidemia), and the $\left[HCO_3^-\right]$ is also lower than normal. Using Winter's formula (Eq. (7.1)), the pCO_2 is consistent with a metabolic acidosis:

$$\begin{aligned} pCO_2 &= 1.5\left[HCO_3^-\right] + 8 \pm 2 \\ &= 1.5 \times 12 + 8 \pm 2 \\ &= 26 \pm 2\,\text{mm Hg} \end{aligned}$$

The negative BE (base deficit) is also agreeable with our diagnosis.

Calculating the *AG* (Eq. (5.2)):

$$\begin{aligned} AG &= \left[Na^+\right] - \left(\left[Cl^-\right] + \left[HCO_3^-\right]\right) \\ &= 140 - (104 + 12) \\ &= 24\,\text{mEq / L} \end{aligned}$$

It can be found that the *AG* is higher than normal (12 ± 2 mEq/L); thus, the patient has a high-*AG* metabolic acidosis. The high-*AG* metabolic acidosis in this patient is due to the release of lactic acid produced by anaerobic metabolism in previously under-perfused tissues. Therefore, this is a *lactic acidosis*.

7.7 Treatment of Metabolic Acidosis

The therapeutic goal should be directed at *removing the underlying problem*, but in severe acidosis ($pH < 7.15$), the administration of bicarbonate is essential [11, 12].

In high-*AG* acidosis, in which unmeasured anions can be metabolized to bicarbonate (e.g., diabetic ketoacidosis or lactic acidosis), correction of the underlying cause (e.g., infusion of saline and insulin in diabetic ketoacidosis (DKA), or increasing peripheral perfusion in lactic acidosis) can alleviate acidosis without any bicarbonate therapy.

Mild metabolic acidosis requires no treatment, except in growing children in whom longstanding acidosis may cause osteomalacia (due to the buffering action of bone) and those with renal tubular acidosis (RTA), to avoid hypercalciuria and its resultant osteomalacia [13].

The required dosage of bicarbonate depends on the degree of acidosis, plasma $\left[HCO_3^-\right]$, and also the underlying cause of acidosis. In order to prevent any complications, the amount of bicarbonate to be administered should be just enough to raise the serum $\left[HCO_3^-\right]$ to 12 mEq/L, and blood *pH* to 7.25. As a rule, the dosage of bicarbonate can be calculated as follows:

$$\left[HCO_3^-\right]_{\text{deficit}} = 0.5\text{Wt}\left(\left[HCO_3^-\right]_{\text{desired}} - \left[HCO_3^-\right]_{\text{measured}}\right) \tag{7.3}$$

where Wt is the body weight in kilogram. Half to whole of the calculated value should be infused intravenously within 3–4 h according to the urgency of the clinical condition. Further alkali replacement must be guided by repeated measurement of serum $\left[HCO_3^-\right]$ and *pH*. Do not forget that *more bicarbonate can always be given*, though once the sodium bicarbonate is in, it cannot be taken out if too much was administered. As a general rule, the sodium bicarbonate to be administered at first should be diluted (usually 2–3 vials of 7.5% $NaHCO_3$ (44.6 mEq in each vial) should be added to 1000 mL of 5% dextrose in water).

As previously mentioned, during alkali therapy, potassium shifts to the intracellular space, thus the *correction of acidosis without supplying the potassium deficit may cause severe hypokalemia and even death*. The management of metabolic acidosis, therefore, includes three steps:

1. Removing the underlying problem.
2. Alkali therapy in severe or symptomatic acidosis:
   (a) oral route
   (b) intravenous infusion of diluted bicarbonate
3. Close monitoring of serum $[K^+]$

Example A 37-year-old woman was hospitalized because of her third episode of nephrolithiasis. Laboratory studies revealed:

Serum electrolytes and chemistries:

$[Na^+] = 133$ mEq/L, $[K^+] = 2.6$ mEq/L, $[Cl^-] = 106$ mEq/L, Calcium: 9.6 mg/dL, Creatinine: 1.1 mg/dL, Albumin: 4.2 mg/dL

Arterial blood:

$pCO_2 = 33$ mm Hg, $\left[HCO_3^-\right] = 16$ mEq/L, $pH = 7.307$, BE = −8.91 mEq/L

Urine $pH = 7.21$

Roentgenography disclosed nephrocalcinosis.

(a) What is your diagnosis?
(b) What happens to plasma $[K^+]$ if arterial *pH* is increased to 7.4?

Solution: Regarding blood *pH* and serum $\left[HCO_3^-\right]$, the patient has acidosis. Using Winter's formula (Eq. (7.1)), the arterial pCO_2 is appropriate for a metabolic acidosis:

$$\begin{aligned} pCO_2 &= 1.5\left[HCO_3^-\right] + 8 \pm 2 \\ &= 1.5 \times 16 + 8 \pm 2 \\ &= 32 \pm 2\,\text{mm Hg} \end{aligned}$$

The negative value of BE (−8.91) is also in favor of our diagnosis. The *AG* is normal (Eq. (5.2)):

$$\begin{aligned} AG &= \left[Na^+\right] - \left(\left[Cl^-\right] + \left[HCO_3^-\right]\right) \\ &= 133 - (106 + 16) \\ &= 11\,\text{mEq / L} \end{aligned}$$

Thus, the patient has a normal-*AG* (hyperchloremic) metabolic acidosis.

This patient, with a history of recurrent episodes of renal calculi and nephrocalcinosis, has a normal serum calcium level. The serum electrolyte pattern is characteristic for distal renal tubular acidosis (type I RTA), a disease in which the patient has a problem in distal tubule acid secretion. The patient has an alkaline urine, with evidence of renal potassium wasting. Thus, the diagnosis is normal-*AG* (hyperchloremic) metabolic acidosis due to distal (type I) RTA.

If the arterial blood *pH* is increased to 7.4 without any potassium supplement, the serum $[K^+]$ drops to 2 mEq/L (Eq. (5.1)):

$$\begin{aligned}\Delta\left[K^+\right] &= -6\Delta pH \\ &= -6\times\left(7.4-7.303\right) \\ &= -0.6\,\text{mEq}/\text{L}\end{aligned}$$

a very low value which would need prompt attention.

Longstanding metabolic acidosis does not require any treatment, but in severe cases (serum $\left[HCO_3^-\right]$ < 12 mEq/L), which may cause osteomalacia, especially in growing children, bicarbonate replacement is mandatory. Prolonged metabolic acidosis, on the one hand, causes mobilization of calcium and phosphate from the bone matrix with resultant depletion of bone minerals and osteomalacia. On the other hand, the prolonged acidosis blocks the conversion of 25-hydroxy cholecalciferol to 1,25-dihydroxy cholecalciferol (the active form of vitamin D), which decreases calcium absorption in the gastrointestinal tract.

7.7.1 Complications of Sodium Bicarbonate Therapy

Rapid administration of sodium bicarbonate may precipitate hypocalcemia and tetany, hypernatremia, hypertension, edema, congestive heart failure (due to volume overload), fatal cardiac arrhythmia, and paradoxical CNS acidosis (bicarbonate cannot cross the blood-brain barrier readily; rapid administration of bicarbonate may correct the blood *pH* but leave the cerebrospinal fluid (CSF) acidotic). Massive bicarbonate therapy may also result in hyperosmolar state (6 mosm/L for each 50 mEq of sodium bicarbonate), increased cerebral vascular resistance, tissue hypoxia (due to leftward shift of oxyhemoglobin dissociation curve), hypernatremia and volume overload, hypokalemia, and pulmonary hypertension.

7.8 Diagnosis of Metabolic Alkalosis

As in other disorders, the first step is a careful history-taking in which the history of vomiting and drug ingestion (e.g., furosemide or thiazide) should be noted. Then, an accurate physical examination, with special attention to any sign of dehydration, Cushingoid face and tetany, should be performed. At last, an arterial blood gas analysis and serum electrolyte should be examined.

As mentioned earlier, a positive base excess implies an excess of base and represents metabolic alkalosis or a compensated respiratory acidosis. Considering the blood *pH*, the diagnosis is obvious. Alkalemia conveys metabolic alkalosis, whereas acidemia represents a compensated respiratory acidosis.

As previously mentioned, the level of respiratory compensation for a metabolic alkalosis depends on many factors such as arterial pO_2 and $[K^+]$. This causes the metabolic alkalosis, rather than other simple acid-base disorders (i.e., respiratory acidosis, respiratory alkalosis, and metabolic acidosis), has a significantly more variable level of respiratory compensation for a given serum $\left[HCO_3^-\right]$. The mean compensatory increase in arterial pCO_2 can be designated as 0.4–0.9 mm Hg for each mEq/L raise in plasma $\left[HCO_3^-\right]$, that is:

$$\Delta pCO_2 = (0.4\,\text{to}\,0.9)\Delta\left[HCO_3^-\right] \tag{7.4}$$

We proposed a simple equation similar to the Winter's formula (Eq. (7.1)) for prediction of the respiratory compensation in metabolic alkalosis [14]:

$$pCO_2 = 0.5\left[HCO_3^-\right] + 28 \pm 4 \tag{7.5}$$

If the measured pCO_2 is significantly lower than the predicted value, then a coexisting respiratory alkalosis should be considered. On the other hand, a measured pCO_2 significantly higher than the predicted value indicates that the respiratory response is out of proportion to the alkalosis, and a respiratory acidosis coexists.

Alkalemia inhibits ventilation in such an extent that may finally lead to hypoxemia. If the arterial pO_2 drops below 65 mm Hg, the respiratory center will be stimulated, thus inhibiting a greater elevation of pCO_2. Therefore, the pCO_2 level, after compensation, rarely exceeds 55 mm Hg, unless a coexisting respiratory acidosis is also present. As in metabolic acidosis, here again a *pH* change after full compensation can be expressed as the following equation:

$$\left[HCO_3^-\right] + 15 \approx 2\,\text{digits after decimal point of blood}\,pH \tag{7.6}$$

Example A 46-year-old man who had a history of duodenal ulcer was admitted to hospital after a 10-day history of repeated episodes of post-prandial vomiting. On examination, blood pressure was 100/70 mm Hg; he was not febrile. Blood gas analysis disclosed:

$pCO_2 = 46$ mm Hg, $\left[HCO_3^-\right] = 37$ mEq/L, $pH = 7.527$, BE = 13.85 mEq/L. What is the most likely diagnosis in this patient?

Solution: The blood *pH* indicates alkalemia, an increased blood level of $\left[HCO_3^-\right]$, and the proportionate rise in pCO_2 are in favor of a metabolic alkalosis (Eq. (7.4)):

$$\begin{aligned}\Delta pCO_2 &= (0.4\,\text{to}\,0.9)\Delta\left[HCO_3^-\right]\\ &= (0.4\,\text{to}\,0.9)\times(37-24)\\ &= (0.4\,\text{to}\,0.9)\times 13\\ &= 5.2\,\text{to}\,11.7\,\text{mm Hg}\end{aligned}$$

Then:

$$\begin{aligned}pCO_2 &= 40+(5.2\,\text{to}\,11.7)\\ &= 45.2\,\text{to}\,51.7\,\text{mm Hg}\end{aligned}$$

The positive BE also does agree with the diagnosis of metabolic alkalosis. It seems that the patient has a pyloric outlet obstruction due to longstanding duodenal ulcer. The produced metabolic alkalosis in this case is because of acid loss by vomiting of acid gastric content. Our proposed formula (Eq. (7.5)) results in similar diagnosis:

$$\begin{aligned}pCO_2 &= 0.5\left[HCO_3^-\right]+28\pm 4\\ &= 0.5\times 37+28\pm 4\\ &= 46.5\pm 4\,\text{mm Hg}\end{aligned}$$

Example A 50-year-old lady with no significant past medical history underwent elective cholecystectomy. She developed post-operative ileus needing prolonged nasogastric intermittent suction. On the 6th post-operative day, the nasogastric tube is still in place. She has a poor skin turgor, dry mucous membranes, and an orthostatic hypotension. The results of laboratory studies are reported as follows:

$pCO_2 = 47$ mm Hg, $\left[HCO_3^-\right] = 40$ mEq/L, $pH = 7.551$, BE = 16.51 mEq/L. What is your diagnosis?

Solution: The alkalemia, with high blood $\left[HCO_3^-\right]$, associated with a harmonious increase in pCO_2, reflect a metabolic alkalosis (Eq. (7.4)):

$$\begin{aligned}\Delta pCO_2 &= (0.4\,\text{to}\,0.9)\Delta\left[HCO_3^-\right]\\ &= (0.4\,\text{to}\,0.9)\times(40-24)\\ &= (0.4\,\text{to}\,0.9)\times 16\\ &= 6.4\,\text{to}\,14.4\,\text{mm Hg}\end{aligned}$$

Then:

$$\begin{aligned}pCO_2 &= 40+(6.4\,\text{to}\,14.4)\\ &= 46.4\,\text{to}\,54.4\,\text{mm Hg}\end{aligned}$$

The positive BE is also in favor of our diagnosis. Eq. (7.5) also confirms the similar diagnosis [14]:

$$
\begin{aligned}
pCO_2 &= 0.5\left[HCO_3^-\right] + 28 \pm 4 \\
&= 0.5 \times 40 + 28 \pm 4 \\
&= 48 \pm 4\,\text{mm Hg}
\end{aligned}
$$

As an interesting point, using Eq. (7.6), we have:

$$
\left[HCO_3^-\right] + 15 \approx 2\,\text{digits after decimal point of blood}\ p\text{H}
$$

$$
40 + 15 = 7.\underline{55}1
$$

Considering the history and physical examination, the patient is dehydrated. In such cases, rehydration per se is usually sufficient to correct the alkalosis.

7.9 Treatment of Metabolic Alkalosis

As in other acid-base disorders, here again the treatment should be directed at removing the underlying cause. A therapeutic classification can be made upon the measured urinary chloride concentration in a spot urine collection in a patient who has not received any diuretic (Table 7.3). If the urinary chloride concentration is less than 10 mEq/L, extracellular volume and chloride depletion (e.g., vomiting, nasogastric suction, and congenital chloride wasting diarrhea) are the most important causes [15]. These patients show good response to the administration of chloride salts and volume expansion. On the other hand, a urinary chloride concentration more than 20 mEq/L indicates either recent use of diuretics, or severe hypokalemia (serum $[K^+] < 2$ mEq/L, a potassium deficit of about 500 mEq), or primary aldosteronism (which stimulates renal retention of $\left[HCO_3^-\right]$ and loss of H^+ ions), and they will therefore have no response to the administration of chloride salts [16].

Table 7.3 Therapeutic classification of metabolic alkalosis

Chloride responsive (Urinary $[Cl^-] < 10$ mEq/L)	Chloride resistant (Urinary $[Cl^-] > 20$ mEq/L)
GI loss	Glucocorticoid excess
Vomiting	Mineralocorticoid excess
Nasogastric suction	Primary reninism
Chloride wasting diarrhea	Bartter's syndrome
Villous adenoma colon	Liddle's syndrome
Exogenous	Hypokalemia
$NaHCO_3$ (baking soda)	Hypercalcemia
Lactate or citrate	Alkali ingestion
Massive transfusion	Refeeding alkalosis
Anti-acid therapy	
Diuretic therapy	
Poorly reabsorbable anion	
Carbenicillin	
Penicillin	

7.9.1 Saline (Chloride) Responsive Alkalosis

A great majority of cases with metabolic alkalosis have an associated volume contraction which stimulates renal $\left[HCO_3^-\right]$, Na^+, and Cl^- reabsorption and H^+ and K^+ wasting, thereby, urinary concentration of Na^+ and Cl^- are low (less than 10 mEq/L) and urinary $[K^+]$ (despite systemic hypokalemia) is high (more than 20 mEq/L). Re-expansion of extracellular fluid increases kidney perfusion and GFR. The distal nephron retains Cl^- and excretes $\left[HCO_3^-\right]$, which results in the correction of metabolic alkalosis [17]. The route of volume expansion depends on the severity of volume contraction. If the patient has mild postural hypotension, oral fluid therapy may be sufficient, but in a patient with moderate to severe hypotension parenteral fluid replacement is indicated. Besides chloride salt replacement and volume expansion, ongoing K^+ losses should also be replaced. In a patient with metabolic alkalosis and congestive heart failure, for which volume expansion (saline administration) is contraindicated, the use of 125–500 mg of acetazolamide (Diamox), that is, a carbonic anhydrase inhibitor, is recommended. In such cases, the administration of K^+ is essential. Acetazolamide also may be used if a primary mineralocorticoid excess (e.g., primary aldosteronism) presents. Cimetidine (Tagamet), an H_2 histamine receptor blocker, may be useful in a patient with persisting nasogastric suction (gastric alkalosis). Cimetidine 300 mg iv q6h decreases acid secretion by the stomach, thus minimizing gastric acid losses [18].

In a patient with renal failure associated with metabolic alkalosis ($pH > 7.5$), although renal failure has an acidifying effect, neuromuscular excitability and cardiotoxicity may be seen. Thus, acid therapy, dialysis, or both are recommended [19]. Ammonium chloride, arginine monohydrochloride, and lysine monohydrochloride are acidifying agents which are metabolized to urea and HCl by the liver. However, they produce azotemia and hyperkalemia, which may worsen the condition.

Bicarbonate can be bounded by ionized calcium in the intestine; therefore, oral (but not parenteral) preparations of calcium chloride are acidifying agents.

The best acidifying effect may be achieved by parenteral HCl, which should be infused via a large central vein as a solution with 100–200 mEq/L, and at an infusion rate of not more than 15–20 mEq per hour. However, this treatment should only be reserved for life-threatening conditions.

7.9.2 Saline (Chloride) Unresponsive Alkalosis

The most common causes of this type of alkalosis include hypokalemia, and mineralocorticoid excess with normal or increased extracellular fluid volume [10, 15]. The treatment in such circumstances includes mineralocorticoid antagonist, Na^+ restriction, and K^+ supplement. The best treatment in mineralocorticoid excess is 300–600 mg spironolactone (Aldactone), a potassium-sparing diuretic, daily. Triamterene (Dyrenium), another potassium-sparing diuretic, 200–300 mg daily may also be useful. The best treatment for adrenal tumors is their surgical excision.

During correction of both saline (chloride) responsive and unresponsive alkalosis, arterial blood gas, *pH*, and electrolytes should be monitored frequently. In particular, the monitoring of serum [K^+] is essential. Serum [K^+] declines by 0.6 (0.3–1.3) mEq/L for each 0.1 unit rise in *pH*, that is:

$$\Delta\left[K^+\right] = -6\Delta pH$$

Example A 21-year-old pregnant woman is hospitalized 2 days after she inserted a metal rod into her uterus during an abortion attempt. She has a temperature of 41 °C, shaking chills, and a purulent malodorous vaginal discharge. Blood pressure is 110/65 mm Hg. Laboratory values reveal:

pCO_2 = 27 mm Hg, $\left[HCO_3^-\right]$ = 13 mEq/L, *pH* = 7.304, BE = −11.68 mEq/L. [Na^+] = 138 mEq/L, [K^+] = 4 mEq/L, [Cl^-] = 102 mEq/L

What is your diagnosis?

Solution: Regarding blood *pH*, $\left[HCO_3^-\right]$, and proportionate change of pCO_2, the patient has a metabolic acidosis. Calculation of the *AG* reveals that the condition is a high-*AG* state (Eq. (5.2)):

$$\begin{aligned} AG &= \left[Na^+\right] + \left(\left[Cl^-\right] + \left[HCO_3^-\right]\right) \\ &= 138 - (102 + 13) \\ &= 23\,\text{mEq}/\text{L} \end{aligned}$$

Therefore, the patient has a high-*AG* metabolic acidosis, and its cause is septic abortion.

Example A 6-year-old boy was hospitalized with a history of 5 days of profuse diarrhea. He was lethargic and had an incoherent response to questions. He had poor skin turgor and sunken eye balls, and was breathing deeply. On examination, the vital signs were as follows:

Rectal temperature: 40 °C, Pulse rate: 117/min, Respiratory rate: 25/min, Blood pressure: 95/65 mm Hg.

Arterial blood gas analysis was reported as:

pCO_2 = 18 mm Hg, $\left[HCO_3^-\right]$ = 6 mEq/L, *pH* = 7.144, BE = −21.10 mEq/L. Other laboratory values disclosed the following data:

[Na^+] = 139 mEq/L, [K^+] = 5.4 mEq/L, [Cl^-] = 120 mEq/L, Hematocrit: 59%.

What is your diagnosis?

Solution: The very low *pH* and $\left[HCO_3^-\right]$ and the proportionate pCO_2 are all consistent with a metabolic acidosis. Calculation of anion gap reveals a normal value of

13 mEq/L. Therefore, the condition is a normal-*AG* (hyperchloremic) metabolic acidosis. In spite of an ample serum [K^+] in this patient, he has a low body potassium content. Careless administration of potassium-free alkaline solutions to such a patient causes shift of extracellular K^+ into cells and precipitates a severe fatal hypokalemia.

Example A 15-year-old girl in a lethargic state was brought to the emergency room. Her mother described that she had become listless during the preceding 12 h and had excreted a large volume of urine. On admission, she appeared rather thin and frail, and had a deep rapid respiration. The vital signs were as follows:

Rectal temperature: 39.7 °C, Pulse rate: 78/min, Respiratory rate: 28/min, Blood pressure: 120/80 mm Hg.

Arterial blood gas analysis was reported as:

$pCO_2 = 21$ mm Hg, $\left[HCO_3^-\right] = 8$ mEq/L, $pH = 7.202$, BE = −17.97 mEq/L. Other laboratory values disclosed the following data:

[Na^+] = 140 mEq/L, [K^+] = 5.8 mEq/L, [Cl^-] = 104 mEq/L,
Glucose: 260 mg/dL, Hematocrit: 45%, Hemoglobin: 15 g/dL
Urinalysis revealed a cloudy urine with 4^+ ketone and 3^+ sugar.
What is your diagnosis?

Solution: The arterial blood gas values indicate a metabolic acidosis. Based upon the blood chemistry, the *AG* in this patient is 28 mEq/L. Such a very high *AG* (> 25 mEq/L) can only be seen in diabetic ketoacidosis (DKA), poisoning with methanol, ethylene glycol, salicylate, or lactic acidosis. Regarding blood glucose concentration, glucosuria, and ketonuria, the diagnosis is clear—DKA with a resultant high-*AG* metabolic acidosis.

Example A 25-year-old boy, who was hurt in a car accident, was hospitalized in a comatose state. He had multiple fractures. Laparotomy was performed and a liver laceration was repaired. To preserve his systolic pressure above 100 mm Hg, he was given a total of 15 units of blood before and during the surgery. His laboratory values were normal pre-operatively, but 12 h post-operatively his arterial blood gas analysis revealed:

$pCO_2 = 50$ mm Hg, $\left[HCO_3^-\right] = 40$ mEq/L, $pH = 7.525$, BE = 16.41 mEq/L. What is your diagnosis? What is responsible for this condition?

Solution: The alkalemia and high blood $\left[HCO_3^-\right]$, and an associated proportionate rise in arterial pCO_2 reflects a metabolic alkalosis (Eq. (7.4)):

$$\begin{aligned}\Delta pCO_2 &= (0.4\,\text{to}\,0.9)\Delta\left[HCO_3^-\right]\\ &= (0.4\,\text{to}\,0.9)\times(40-24)\\ &= (0.4\,\text{to}\,0.9)\times 16\\ &= 6.4\,\text{to}\,14.4\,\text{mm Hg}\end{aligned}$$

Then:

$$pCO_2 = 40 + (6.4 \text{ to } 14.4)$$
$$= 46.4 \text{ to } 54.4 \text{ mm Hg}$$

Equation (7.5) also confirms the same diagnosis:

$$pCO_2 = 0.5\left[HCO_3^-\right] + 28 \pm 4$$
$$= 0.5 \times 40 + 28 \pm 4$$
$$= 48 \pm 4 \text{ mm Hg}$$

The positive BE (16.41 mEq/L) is consistent with our diagnosis too. The metabolic alkalosis in this case is because of the citrate load from massive blood transfusion.

Example A 15-year-old girl was admitted to the ICU due to Guillain-Barré syndrome. The muscular weakness was generalized and respiratory muscles were also involved, thus an endotracheal tube was inserted and mechanical ventilation was started. On the third day, her arterial blood gas values disclosed the following data:

pCO_2 = 55 mm Hg, $\left[HCO_3^-\right]$ = 29 mEq/L, pH = 7.343, BE = 2.60 mEq/L. For lowering the high pCO_2, the on-call intern increased the respiratory rate. Twenty minutes later, another blood gas analysis was reported as:

pCO_2 = 37 mm Hg, $\left[HCO_3^-\right]$ = 28.9 mEq/L, pH = 7.514, BE = 6.69 mEq/L. What happened to this patient?

Solution: The first arterial blood gas data reveal a chronic respiratory acidosis (Eq. (6.2)):

$$\Delta\left[HCO_3^-\right] = 0.4\Delta pCO_2 \pm 2$$
$$= 0.4 \times (55 - 40) \pm 2$$
$$= 6 \pm 2 \text{ mEq / L}$$

The second blood gas data indicate a high pH (7.514), $\left[HCO_3^-\right]$ (28.9 mEq/L), and BE (6.69 mEq/L), typical for a metabolic alkalosis.

$$\Delta pCO_2 = (0.4 \text{ to } 0.9)\Delta\left[HCO_3^-\right]$$
$$= (0.4 \text{ to } 0.9) \times (28.9 - 24)$$
$$= (0.4 \text{ to } 0.9) \times 4.9$$
$$= 1.96 \text{ to } 4.41 \text{ mm Hg}$$

Then:

$$pCO_2 = 40 + (1.96 \text{ to } 4.41)$$
$$= 41.96 \text{ to } 44.41 \text{ mm Hg}$$

The measured pCO_2 is lower than that expected (without using Eq. (7.4), it is also obvious that the pCO_2 is not proportionate, and is even lower than 40 mm Hg). What happened? Is there any superimposed respiratory alkalosis over a metabolic alkalosis? The answer is NO! At first, the patient had a well-compensated (chronic) respiratory acidosis. The pCO_2 was accumulated and the body responded to this hypercapnia by reabsorption and the generation of new bicarbonate and increased serum $\left[HCO_3^-\right]$. Then, after increasing the respiratory rate, the surplus CO_2 was removed rapidly, as reflected by a rapid drop in pCO_2 from 55 to 37 mm Hg, but the serum $\left[HCO_3^-\right]$ could not show such a fast decline (it decreased only from 29 to 28.9 mEq/L). The bicarbonate ions which once acted as a buffer, behaved as an alkaline load and resulted in metabolic alkalosis. In such an acute condition, results obtained from Eqs. (7.4) and (7.5) are wrong (as you have seen in this case). Equations (7.1), (7.4), and (7.5) *can only be used after full compensation*; before that time, they cause wrong interpretation. Therefore, the patient had a *post-hypercapnic metabolic alkalosis*.

7.10 Things to Remember

Any factor that primarily changes the blood $\left[HCO_3^-\right]$ produces a metabolic acid-base disturbance. The causes which decrease the serum $\left[HCO_3^-\right]$, precipitate metabolic acidosis (Table 7.1), whereas those which elevate plasma $\left[HCO_3^-\right]$ cause metabolic alkalosis (Table 7.2). Considering the *AG*, the metabolic acidosis can be categorized into two subgroups: normal-*AG* (hyperchloremic) and high-*AG* metabolic acidosis. Recognition of these subgroups provides an important framework facilitating the diagnosis. For example, as a general rule an unexplained high-*AG* acidosis should suggest sepsis unless proved otherwise; this is because the lactic acidosis secondary to sepsis may be difficult to detect.

The body responds to metabolic disturbances by (1) cellular buffering, (2) adjustment of respiratory drive to alter pCO_2 in such a way that normal *pH* is re-established, and (3) control of kidney acid excretion and new bicarbonate synthesis.

Hypovolemia is a major cause of metabolic alkalosis. In such circumstances, the kidney sacrifice body fluid tonicity and acid-base balance to preserve volume; that is, in spite of hyperbicarbonatemia, it may reabsorb $NaHCO_3$. Thus, in metabolic alkalosis the kidney may react in another way.

Regarding blood *pH*, pCO_2, $\left[HCO_3^-\right]$, BE, history, and physical examination, the diagnosis of metabolic acidosis is simple (Table 7.4). The treatment of metabolic acidosis includes treatment of the underlying disease and, in severe acidemic cases, bicarbonate therapy.

Based on clinical findings, the patients with metabolic alkalosis can be grouped into two different classes: (1) saline (chloride) responsive, and (2) saline (chloride) unresponsive (Table 7.3). Here again, considering blood *pH*, pCO_2, $\left[HCO_3^-\right]$, BE, history, and physical examination, the diagnosis is easy (Table 7.4). The treatment

Table 7.4 Changes in blood chemistry in metabolic acid-base disorders

Condition	*pH*	pCO_2	$[HCO_3^-]$	BE
Met. Ac.	$\downarrow$	$\downarrow$: $pCO_2 = 1.5[HCO_3^-] + 8 \pm 2$	$\downarrow$	<−2
Met. Al.	$\uparrow$	$\uparrow$: $\Delta pCO_2 = (0.4 \text{ to } 0.9)\Delta[HCO_3^-]$	$\uparrow$	>2
		$\uparrow$: $pCO_2 = 0.5[HCO_3^-] + 28 \pm 4$		

Met. Ac. Metabolic acidosis, Met. Al. Metabolic alkalosis

should include removing the underlying disease, preserving fluid and electrolyte balance and, in severely ill patients, infusion of acidifying agent (HCl).

The above equations (Eqs. (7.1), (7.4), and (7.5)) can only be used after full compensation; before that, they will lead to the wrong interpretation of the acid-base status.

References

1. DuBose TD Jr. Clinical approach to patients with acid-base disorders. Med Clin North Am. 1983;67(4):799–813. https://doi.org/10.1016/s0025-7125(16)31178-6.
2. Mustaqeem R, Arif A. Renal tubular acidosis. Treasure Island, FL: StatPearls; 2020.
3. Goraya N, Wesson DE. Management of the metabolic acidosis of chronic kidney disease. Adv Chronic Kidney Dis. 2017;24(5):298–304. https://doi.org/10.1053/j.ackd.2017.06.006.
4. Kraut JA, Madias NE. Adverse effects of the metabolic acidosis of chronic kidney disease. Adv Chronic Kidney Dis. 2017;24(5):289–97. https://doi.org/10.1053/j.ackd.2017.06.005.
5. Berend K. Review of the diagnostic evaluation of Normal anion gap metabolic acidosis. Kidney Dis (Basel). 2017;3(4):149–59. https://doi.org/10.1159/000479279.
6. Brubaker RH, Vashisht R, Meseeha M. High anion gap metabolic acidosis. Treasure Island (FL): StatPearls; 2020.
7. Leclercq F, Leclercq B. Hypokalemic metabolic alkalosis. Treasure Island, FL: StatPearls; 2020.
8. Soifer JT, Kim HT. Approach to metabolic alkalosis. Emerg Med Clin North Am. 2014;32(2):453–63. https://doi.org/10.1016/j.emc.2014.01.005.
9. Szaflarski N, Hanson CW 3rd. Metabolic acidosis. AACN Clin Issues. 1997;8(3):481–96. https://doi.org/10.1097/00044067-199708000-00016.
10. Khanna A, Kurtzman NA. Metabolic alkalosis. J Nephrol. 2006;19(Suppl 9):S86–96.
11. Jung B, Martinez M, Claessens YE, Darmon M, Klouche K, Lautrette A, et al. Diagnosis and management of metabolic acidosis: guidelines from a French expert panel. Ann Intensive Care. 2019;9(1):92. https://doi.org/10.1186/s13613-019-0563-2.
12. Matyukhin I, Patschan S, Ritter O, Patschan D. Etiology and management of acute metabolic acidosis: an update. Kidney Blood Press Res. 2020;45(4):523–31. https://doi.org/10.1159/000507813.
13. Andrade OV, Ihara FO, Troster EJ. Metabolic acidosis in childhood: why, when and how to treat. J Pediatr. 2007;83(2 Suppl):S11–21. https://doi.org/10.2223/JPED.1616.
14. Habibzadeh F, Yadollahie M. Mathematical equivalent of metabolic alkalosis part of the Goldberg acid-base map. Anesthesiology. 1999;91(6):1967. https://doi.org/10.1097/00000542-199912000-00062.

15. Pahari DK, Kazmi W, Raman G, Biswas S. Diagnosis and management of metabolic alkalosis. J Indian Med Assoc. 2006;104(11):630–4. 6
16. Koch SM, Taylor RW. Chloride ion in intensive care medicine. Crit Care Med. 1992;20(2):227–40. https://doi.org/10.1097/00003246-199202000-00012.
17. Hyneck ML. Simple acid-base disorders. Am J Hosp Pharm. 1985;42(9):1992–2004.
18. Banieghbal B. Rapid correction of metabolic alkalosis in hypertrophic pyloric stenosis with intravenous cimetidine: preliminary results. Pediatr Surg Int. 2009;25(3):269–71. https://doi.org/10.1007/s00383-009-2335-9.
19. Martin WJ, Matzke GR. Treating severe metabolic alkalosis. Clin Pharm. 1982;1(1):42–8.

Mixed Disorders

8

8.1 Introduction and Diagnostic Procedures

A primary change in plasma bicarbonate concentration produces a metabolic disturbance (Chapter 7); a primary alteration in pCO_2 causes a respiratory one (Chapter 6). Acidosis is characterized by either a low serum $\left[HCO_3^-\right]$ or a high arterial pCO_2. Contrarily, alkalosis is identified by either a high plasma $\left[HCO_3^-\right]$ or a low arterial pCO_2. Respiratory disorders primarily alter the pCO_2 which in turn changes the ratio $\left[HCO_3^-\right]/(\alpha\, pCO_2)$ in the well-known Henderson-Hasselbalch equation. A secondary change in serum $\left[HCO_3^-\right]$ is needed (compensation) to balance the ratio toward normal. The same processes may occur in metabolic disorders; a primary change in plasma $\left[HCO_3^-\right]$ is followed by a compensatory change in pCO_2. Therefore, after a primary disturbance, a secondary or compensatory change will occur. Such compensatory mechanisms include secondary changes in pCO_2 or serum $\left[HCO_3^-\right]$ for metabolic or respiratory abnormalities, respectively. The failure to compensate normally or the coexistence of two or more simple acid-base disturbances generates a *mixed condition.*

In previous chapters, the compensatory processes, their time course, and limit of compensation were discussed in detail. A summary can be found in Table 8.1.

8.2 Clinical Approach to Mixed Acid-Base Disorders

As previously mentioned, the first and the most important step in interpretation of acid-base status is a careful history-taking, including history of vomiting, diarrhea, trauma, drug ingestion, dyspnea, renal disease, COPD, and asthma.

The second step is a complete physical examination. It might either confirm a suspected diagnosis or suggest a new one. For example, deep rapid breathing

F. Habibzadeh et al., *Pathophysiologic Basis of Acid-Base Disorders*,
https://doi.org/10.1007/978-981-16-0526-0_8

Table 8.1 Normal compensation in simple acid-base disturbances

Condition	Primary disturbance	Compensatory response	BE	Clinical guide for compensation	Limit of compensation	Duration required for compensation
Met. Ac.	$\downarrow\downarrow\downarrow\left[HCO_3^-\right]$	$\downarrow\downarrow pCO_2$	<−2	$pCO_2 = 1.5\left[HCO_3^-\right] + 8 \pm 2$	$pCO_2 > 10$ mm Hg	12–24 h
Met. Al.	$\uparrow\uparrow\uparrow\left[HCO_3^-\right]$	$\uparrow\uparrow pCO_2$	>2	$pCO_2 = 0.5\left[HCO_3^-\right] + 28 \pm 4$	$pCO_2 < 55$ mm Hg	12–24 h
				$\Delta pCO_2 = (0.4 \text{ to } 0.9)\,\Delta\left[HCO_3^-\right]$		
Acute R. Ac.	$\uparrow\uparrow\uparrow pCO_2$	$\uparrow\left[HCO_3^-\right]$	Nl	$\Delta\left[HCO_3^-\right] = 0.1\,\Delta pCO_2$	$\left[HCO_3^-\right] < 30$ mEq/L	Within minutes
Chronic R. Ac.	$\uparrow\uparrow\uparrow pCO_2$	$\uparrow\uparrow\left[HCO_3^-\right]$	>2	$\Delta\left[HCO_3^-\right] = 0.4\,\Delta pCO_2$	$\left[HCO_3^-\right] < 45$ mEq/L	3–5 days
Acute R. Al.	$\downarrow\downarrow\downarrow pCO_2$	$\downarrow\left[HCO_3^-\right]$	Nl	$\Delta\left[HCO_3^-\right] = 0.2\,\Delta pCO_2$	$\left[HCO_3^-\right] > 18$ mEq/L	Within minutes
Chronic R. Al.	$\downarrow\downarrow\downarrow pCO_2$	$\downarrow\downarrow\left[HCO_3^-\right]$	<−2	$\Delta\left[HCO_3^-\right] = 0.5\,\Delta pCO_2$	$\left[HCO_3^-\right] > 12$ mEq/L	2–3 days

Met. Metabolic, R. Respiratory, Ac. Acidosis, Al. Alkalosis, Nl Normal

(Kussmaul's respiration) suggests a metabolic acidosis, and any sign of dehydration reflects a metabolic alkalosis.

The third step is to perform some laboratory examinations which may support or oppose the acid-base disturbance that was expected considering the data found in history and physical examination. Examples of such studies are measurement of serum $\left[HCO_3^-\right]$, $[K^+]$, $[Na^+]$, $[Cl^-]$ for the calculation of the anion gap (*AG*); serum creatinine concentration for determination of renal function, whose failure may be associated with a metabolic acidosis; blood glucose and serum ketone concentrations for the diagnosis of diabetic ketoacidosis; and so on.

The change in serum $[K^+]$ is much more significant in metabolic than in respiratory disorders. A low serum $\left[HCO_3^-\right]$ associated with hyperkalemia implies a metabolic acidosis, whereas a high serum $\left[HCO_3^-\right]$ associated with hypokalemia (shift of extracellular K^+) proposes a metabolic alkalosis. A low serum $[Cl^-]$ indicates either a metabolic alkalosis or a respiratory acidosis, whereas a high serum $[Cl^-]$ associated with a low plasma $\left[HCO_3^-\right]$ may reflect either a hyperchloremic metabolic acidosis or a compensated respiratory alkalosis. A serum $\left[HCO_3^-\right]$ of less than 12 mEq/L indicates a metabolic acidosis since metabolic compensation of chronic respiratory alkalosis rarely reduces the plasma $\left[HCO_3^-\right]$ less than 12 mEq/L. Similarly, a serum $\left[HCO_3^-\right]$ of more than 45 mEq/L usually implies a metabolic alkalosis since metabolic compensation of chronic respiratory acidosis seldom elevates the plasma $\left[HCO_3^-\right]$ to such an extent. Finally, calculation of the *AG* may be helpful in diagnosing and managing the disease. As presented previously, the *AG* is the amount of unmeasurable anions in the plasma and is usually calculated as follows:

$$AG = \left[Na^+\right] - \left(\left[Cl^-\right] + \left[HCO_3^-\right]\right)$$

The normal value of the *AG* is 12 ± 2 mmol/L. A low serum $\left[HCO_3^-\right]$ may be associated with a high-*AG* metabolic acidosis, but a high *AG*, regardless of the serum $\left[HCO_3^-\right]$, indicates a metabolic acidosis. If each mmol of the lost $\left[HCO_3^-\right]$ is replaced by an equal amount of Cl^-, then a normal-*AG* (hyperchloremic) acidosis will be produced. In a simple (not mixed) high-*AG* acidosis, the fall in serum bicarbonate concentration $\left(\Delta\left[HCO_3^-\right]\right)$ should be just equal to the rise in the *AG* (ΔAG). If ΔAG exceeds $\Delta\left[HCO_3^-\right]$, some alkali (e.g., by vomiting, or diuretics) must have been added to the body fluids. This causes a mixed metabolic acidosis and metabolic alkalosis. Conversely, a ΔAG lesser than $\Delta\left[HCO_3^-\right]$ implies the coexistence of a normal and a high-*AG* metabolic acidosis.

In mixed acid-base conditions, the final blood *pH* reflects the dominant pathologic process. Do not forget that even *a normal pH does not rule out the presence of a mixed disturbance* since the processes may cancel out the effect of each other on the plasma *pH*, but they usually change the serum chemistry. A normal *pH* with an abnormal $\left[HCO_3^-\right]$ or pCO_2 is highly suggestive of a mixed problem since the *compensatory mechanisms rarely tend to return the blood pH to normal.* Besides all of these laboratory measurements, an arterial blood gas analysis (e.g., pO_2) may be needed.

Finally, the predicted compensatory response including its magnitude and time course must be noted (Table 8.1). As an example, in metabolic acidosis complete respiratory compensation takes 12–24 h, and the pCO_2, even in the worst condition, rarely drops to a value lesser than 10 mm Hg. If the predicted compensatory level differs significantly from those measured, the patient should have a mixed acid-base disorder.

Base excess (BE) and serum $\left[HCO_3^-\right]$ are good guidelines for rapid assessment of arterial blood gas data. A positive BE or a high serum $\left[HCO_3^-\right]$ indicates either a metabolic alkalosis or a compensated respiratory acidosis, whereas a negative BE or a low $\left[HCO_3^-\right]$ implies either a metabolic acidosis or a compensated respiratory alkalosis. The diagnosis is clear regarding the blood *pH*. In metabolic acidosis or compensated respiratory acidosis, blood *pH* is less than normal (acidemia); on the contrary, in metabolic alkalosis or compensated respiratory alkalosis, blood *pH* is higher than normal (alkalemia).

On some occasions, the acid-base and blood gas data are compatible with more than one diagnosis. In such conditions, the best final diagnosis may be obtained from re-evaluation of the history, physical examination, and paraclinical findings.

8.3 Mixed Acid-Base Disorders

Combination of two or more simple acid-base disorders produces a mixed acid-base disturbance which can be categorized as follows (Table 8.2). The following section explains the most important mixed acid-base disorders.

8.3.1 Mixed Metabolic and Respiratory Acidosis

A primary decrease in plasma $\left[HCO_3^-\right]$ produces metabolic acidosis. The consequent acidification of extracellular fluid stimulates the respiratory center and causes hyperventilation. As already mentioned, the predicted value for the respiratory compensation may be calculated by Winter's formula:

$$pCO_2 = 1.5\left[HCO_3^-\right] + 8 \pm 2 \qquad (7.1)$$

If the measured arterial pCO_2 is significantly higher than the predicted value, a mixed metabolic and respiratory acidosis must be considered [1, 2].

Example A 47-year-old man, also with chronic emphysema, was admitted to the hospital with profuse watery diarrhea of 4 days duration. On admission, his arterial blood gas analysis gave the following values:

$pCO_2 = 47$ mm Hg, $\left[HCO_3^-\right] = 18$ mEq/L, $pH = 7.205$, BE = −8.87 mEq/L. The serum chemistry reveals:

$[Na^+] = 137$ mEq/L, $[K^+] = 4.7$ mEq/L, $[Cl^-] = 100$ mEq/L

What is your diagnosis?

Table 8.2 Classification of the mixed acid-base disorders

Mixed disorder	Example
A. Mixed metabolic acidosis and respiratory acidosis	Cardiopulmonary arrest + resuscitation; severe pulmonary edema; hypoxia + COPD; diarrhea + hypokalemic myopathy; phosphorus depletion; poisoning and drug over-dosage
B. Mixed metabolic acidosis and respiratory alkalosis	Salicylate intoxication; severe liver disease; pulmonary embolism; septic shock in critically ill patients; renal failure + sepsis
C. Mixed metabolic acidosis	
1. Mixed hyperchloremic and high-*AG* metabolic acidosis ($\Delta AG < \Delta\left[HCO_3^-\right]$)	
a. Renal causes	Early chronic renal failure; uremic acidosis + proximal or distal renal tubular acidosis (RTA); interstitial renal disease
b. Extra-renal causes	Diarrhea + diabetic ketoacidosis (DKA)
2. Mixed high-*AG* metabolic acidosis $\left(\Delta AG = \Delta\left[HCO_3^-\right]\right)$	Glycogen storage disease; alcoholic acidosis; toxicity
3. Mixed hyperchloremic metabolic acidosis ($\Delta AG = 0$)	RTA + advanced liver disease; RTA + diarrhea or pancreatitis
D. Mixed metabolic acidosis and alkalosis	Diarrhea + vomiting; renal failure + vomiting; hypotension (lactic acidosis) + vomiting; alcoholic ketoacidosis + vomiting; metabolic acidosis + overshoot metabolic alkalosis
E. Mixed metabolic alkalosis and respiratory acidosis	Diuretic therapy + COPD
F. Mixed metabolic and respiratory alkalosis	Critically ill surgical patient; massive blood transfusion; pregnancy (high progesterone level); misuse of ventilators (overventilation) + nasogastric suction; hepatic failure + diuretic therapy
G. Mixed acute and chronic respiratory acidosis	COPD + superimposed pneumonia
H. Mixed acute and chronic respiratory alkalosis	Severe anemia + CO poisoning; pregnancy + salicylate intoxication
I. Triple acid–base disorders	
1. Mixed metabolic acidosis + metabolic alkalosis + respiratory acidosis	DKA + vomiting + COPD; hypovolemic shock + massive transfusion + pneumothorax
2. Mixed metabolic acidosis + metabolic alkalosis + respiratory alkalosis	DKA + dehydration + fever

Solution: The coexistence of acidemia and low serum $\left[HCO_3^-\right]$ reflects a metabolic acidosis. Employing Winter's formula, we have:

$$\begin{aligned} pCO_2 &= 1.5\left[HCO_3^-\right] + 8 \pm 2 \\ &= 1.5 \times 18 + 8 \pm 2 \\ &= 35 \pm 2\,\text{mEq/L} \end{aligned}$$

But the measured pCO_2 (47 mm Hg) is significantly higher than 37 mm Hg, thus, there should also be a coexistent respiratory acidosis. Therefore, the diagnosis is *mixed metabolic and respiratory acidosis*. The respiratory component is because of chronic emphysema, and the metabolic component is due to prolonged GI bicarbonate loss (what is the type of the metabolic acidosis (high-*AG* or hyperchloremic)?).

Another approach to this patient is considering acidemia and hypercapnia, which means a respiratory acidosis (consistent with the history of lung disease). The compensated bicarbonate, whether in acute or chronic respiratory acidosis, should be greater than 24 mEq/L. The moderately low serum $\left[HCO_3^-\right]$ (18 mEq/L) in this patient reflects the coexistence of a metabolic acidosis. Therefore, the diagnosis is again mixed metabolic and respiratory acidosis.

In mixed metabolic and respiratory acidosis, although the values of serum $\left[HCO_3^-\right]$ and pCO_2 depend on the algebraic sum of each components of the acidosis, severe acidemia is presented (Table 8.3).

In a patient with acidosis, potassium shifts out from the intracellular space in exchange for extracellular H^+; thus, the serum $[K^+]$ is usually high. Therefore, low or low-normal serum potassium concentration indicates severe potassium deficiency, which may even result in muscle paralysis. The respiratory muscle dysfunction finally results in a respiratory acidosis, and the patient develops a mixed

Table 8.3 Blood gas values in mixed metabolic and respiratory acidosis

Condition	*pH*	pCO_2	$\left[HCO_3^-\right]$	BE	Comment
Met. Ac.	↓	↓	↓	–	$pCO_2 = 1.5\left[HCO_3^-\right] + 8 \pm 2$ $> 10\,\text{mm Hg}$
Mixed Met. + R. Ac.	↓↓	?	?	?	$pCO_2 >$ Predicted value or $\left[HCO_3^-\right] <$ Predicted value
R. Ac.	↓	↑	↑	+	$\Delta\left[HCO_3^-\right]_{\text{Acute}} = 0.1\,\Delta pCO_2 \pm 2$ $\left[HCO_3^-\right] < 30\,\text{mEq/L}$ $\Delta\left[HCO_3^-\right]_{\text{Chronic}} = 0.4\,\Delta pCO_2 \pm 2$ $\left[HCO_3^-\right] < 45\,\text{mEq/L}$

Met. Metabolic, R. Respiratory, Ac. Acidosis, ? Unpredictable—low, normal, or high metabolic and respiratory acidosis. Mixed metabolic and respiratory acidosis may be seen in cardiopulmonary arrest, severe pulmonary edema, or toxicity with certain materials such as methanol.

A primary increase in pCO_2 produces respiratory acidosis followed by a compensatory hyperbicarbonatemia. The amount of compensatory change in serum $\left[HCO_3^-\right]$, as was mentioned earlier, is 1 mEq/L for each 10 mm Hg increase in pCO_2 $\left(\Delta\left[HCO_3^-\right] = 0.1\,\Delta pCO_2\right)$, up to a maximum rise of 3–4 mEq/L $\left(\left[HCO_3^-\right] < 30\,mEq/L\right)$ in acute phase, and 4 mEq/L for each 10 mm Hg elevation of pCO_2 $\left(\Delta\left[HCO_3^-\right] = 0.4\,\Delta pCO_2\right)$, up to a maximum rise of 20 mEq/L $\left(\left[HCO_3^-\right] < 45\,mEq/L\right)$ in chronic phase. A plasma $\left[HCO_3^-\right]$ lower than the predicted value is indicative of a coexisting metabolic acidosis. Thus, in a patient with suspected chronic respiratory acidosis, the predicted $\left[HCO_3^-\right]$ should be calculated; if the measured serum $\left[HCO_3^-\right]$ is lower than the predicted value, then a mixed metabolic and respiratory acidosis must be present.

8.3.1.1 Treatment

The proper management includes simultaneous intensive treatment of both metabolic and respiratory acidosis. At first, the underlying cause of acidemia must be corrected (e.g., correction of tissue perfusion in a patient with hypotension). In a hypoxic ($p_aO_2 < 50$ mm Hg) hypercapnic ($p_aCO_2 > 50$ mm Hg) patient (e.g., a hypotensive patient with respiratory failure), oxygen therapy without any ventilatory support (artificial respiration) may increase hypercapnia; the hypoxia-mediated central respiratory drive is diminished. Thus, oxygen should be given in conjunction with artificial ventilatory support. Thereby, in cardiopulmonary arrest, the existing acidemia must be corrected with intravenous infusion of bicarbonate (for alleviation of metabolic acidosis). Meanwhile, artificial respiration should also be initiated (for correction of respiratory acidosis). It should be noted that raising the *pH* by administration of bicarbonate, without any ventilatory support, decreases the acidemia-induced respiratory drive, thus worsens the respiratory component of the acidosis. Consequently, the treatment should be aimed at simultaneous removal of both respiratory and metabolic components.

8.3.2 Mixed Metabolic Acidosis and Respiratory Alkalosis

A primary decrease in serum $\left[HCO_3^-\right]$ produces a metabolic acidosis, which is compensated with a consequent hypocapnia (Eq. (7.1)). A pCO_2 lower than the predicted value reveals a mixed metabolic acidosis and respiratory alkalosis [1, 2].

A primary decrement in pCO_2 causes a respiratory alkalosis which is compensated by a consequent hypobicarbonatemia. A plasma $\left[HCO_3^-\right]$ lower than the predicted value (Eqs. (6.3) and (6.4)) indicates a coexistent metabolic acidosis; hence, a mixed metabolic acidosis and respiratory alkalosis is present.

Table 8.4 Blood gas values in mixed metabolic acidosis and respiratory alkalosis

Condition	*pH*	pCO_2	$[HCO_3^-]$	BE	Comment
Met. Ac.	↓	↓	↓	–	$pCO_2 = 1.5[HCO_3^-] + 8 \pm 2$ > 10 mm Hg
Mixed Met. Ac. + R. Al.	?	↓↓	↓↓	–	$pCO_2 <$ Predicted value or $[HCO_3^-] <$ Predicted value
R. Al.	↑	↓	↓	–	$\Delta[HCO_3^-]_{Acute} = 0.2\,\Delta pCO_2 \pm 2$ $[HCO_3^-] > 18$ mEq/L $\Delta[HCO_3^-]_{Chronic} = 0.5\,\Delta pCO_2 \pm 2$ $[HCO_3^-] > 12$ mEq/L

Met. Metabolic, R. Respiratory, Ac. Acidosis, Al. Alkalosis, ? Unpredictable—low, normal, or high

Mixed metabolic acidosis and respiratory alkalosis can produce a high, low, or even normal *pH*, depending on the severity of metabolic or respiratory components (Table 8.4). Both serum bicarbonate and arterial pCO_2 are very low and associated with moderate hypokalemia.

Anion gap may be increased in metabolic acidosis; therefore, an elevated *AG* accompanied by an alkaline *pH* indicates a mixed disturbance (i.e., mixed high-*AG* metabolic acidosis and respiratory alkalosis).

Example A 25-year-old woman was brought to the emergency room after a suicide attempt. She had reportedly swallowed a handful of pills. On arrival, she complains of shortness of breath and tinnitus, but cannot name the pills she had ingested. Pertinent laboratory values are given below:

$pCO_2 = 11$ mm Hg, $[HCO_3^-] = 8$ mEq/L, $pH = 7.483$, BE = −11.13 mEq/L.

The serum chemistry reveals:

$[Na^+] = 139$ mEq/L, $[K^+] = 4.7$ mEq/L, $[Cl^-] = 103$ mEq/L.

What is the most probable diagnosis?

Solution: The coexistence of alkalemia and hypocapnia indicates a respiratory alkalosis. Then, the expected serum $[HCO_3^-]$ may be calculated as:

If acute:

$$\begin{aligned}\Delta[HCO_3^-] &= 0.2\,\Delta pCO_2 \pm 2 \\ &= 0.2 \times (40 - 11) \pm 2 \\ &= 5.8 \pm 2\,\text{mEq/L}\end{aligned}$$

If chronic:

$$\begin{aligned}\Delta\left[\mathrm{HCO}_3^-\right] &= 0.5\ \Delta p\mathrm{CO}_2 \pm 2\\ &= 0.5\times(40-11)\pm 2\\ &= 14.5\pm 2\,\mathrm{mEq/L}\end{aligned}$$

If the process is acute, the expected serum $\left[\mathrm{HCO}_3^-\right]$ should be about 18.2 ± 2 (= 24–5.8 ± 2) mEq/L; if chronic, the expected $\left[\mathrm{HCO}_3^-\right]$ must be about 9.5 ± 2 (= 24–14.5 ± 2) mEq/L. The measured serum $\left[\mathrm{HCO}_3^-\right]$ (8 mEq/L) is compatible with a chronic respiratory alkalosis and is very much lower than the predicted value for an acute respiratory alkalosis. Therefore, the diagnosis may be either *a chronic respiratory alkalosis*, or *a mixed acute respiratory alkalosis and metabolic acidosis*. Calculating the *AG*, we have:

$$\begin{aligned}AG &= \left[\mathrm{Na}^+\right]-\left(\left[\mathrm{Cl}^-\right]+\left[\mathrm{HCO}_3^-\right]\right)\\ &= 139-(103+8)\\ &= 28\,\mathrm{mEq/L}\end{aligned}$$

This very high *AG* cannot occur in a simple chronic respiratory alkalosis and is more in favor of a metabolic acidosis. On the other hand, the history of the patient is also not compatible with a chronic well-compensated process. Thus, the final diagnosis is *mixed acute respiratory alkalosis and high-AG metabolic acidosis*. Actually, all these findings are in favor of salicylate intoxication [3]. Salicylate directly stimulates the medullary respiratory center, causing respiratory alkalosis. Salicylate also produces a concomitant high-*AG* metabolic acidosis due to the accumulation of organic acids. Methanol poisoning can also cause a high-*AG* metabolic acidosis, but without the concomitant respiratory alkalosis. In our patient, the history of tinnitus accompanying mixed respiratory alkalosis and metabolic acidosis, is basically pathognomonic of salicylate intoxication.

8.3.2.1 Treatment

Since blood *pH* is normal, no immediate therapy is required. Treatment should be aimed at correcting the underlying cause. Alkali therapy (e.g., giving sodium bicarbonate) may result in severe alkalemia and is contraindicated.

8.3.3 Mixed Metabolic Acidosis

In a metabolic acidosis, if the decreased serum $\left[\mathrm{HCO}_3^-\right]$ is replaced by chloride, the anion gap remains unchanged; therefore, a normal anion gap or hyperchloremic metabolic acidosis is produced. On the other hand, in a high-*AG* acidosis, bicarbonate is replaced by organic acids such as phosphate and sulfate, i.e., with anions other than Cl^- which cannot be measured easily [4].

8.3.3.1 Mixed Hyperchloremic (Normal-*AG*) and High-*AG* Metabolic Acidosis $\left(\Delta AG < \Delta\left[\mathrm{HCO}_3^-\right]\right)$

In a mixed high- and normal-*AG* acidosis (Fig. 8.1), the decrement in serum $\left[\mathrm{HCO}_3^-\right]$ is partly reflected by the increment in *AG*, and partly by the change in serum [Cl⁻], that is:

$$\begin{array}{rl} \text{Normal } AG & : \Delta\left[\mathrm{HCO}_3^-\right] = \Delta\left[\mathrm{Cl}^-\right] \\ +\,\text{High } AG & : \Delta\left[\mathrm{HCO}_3^-\right] = \Delta AG \\ \hline (\text{Normal} + \text{High})\, AG & : \Delta\left[\mathrm{HCO}_3^-\right] = \Delta AG + \Delta\left[\mathrm{Cl}^-\right] \end{array}$$

thus, the serum electrolyte composition should be used as a diagnostic aid. In general, we have:

$$\Delta\left[\mathrm{HCO}_3^-\right] = \Delta AG + \Delta\left[\mathrm{Cl}^-\right]$$

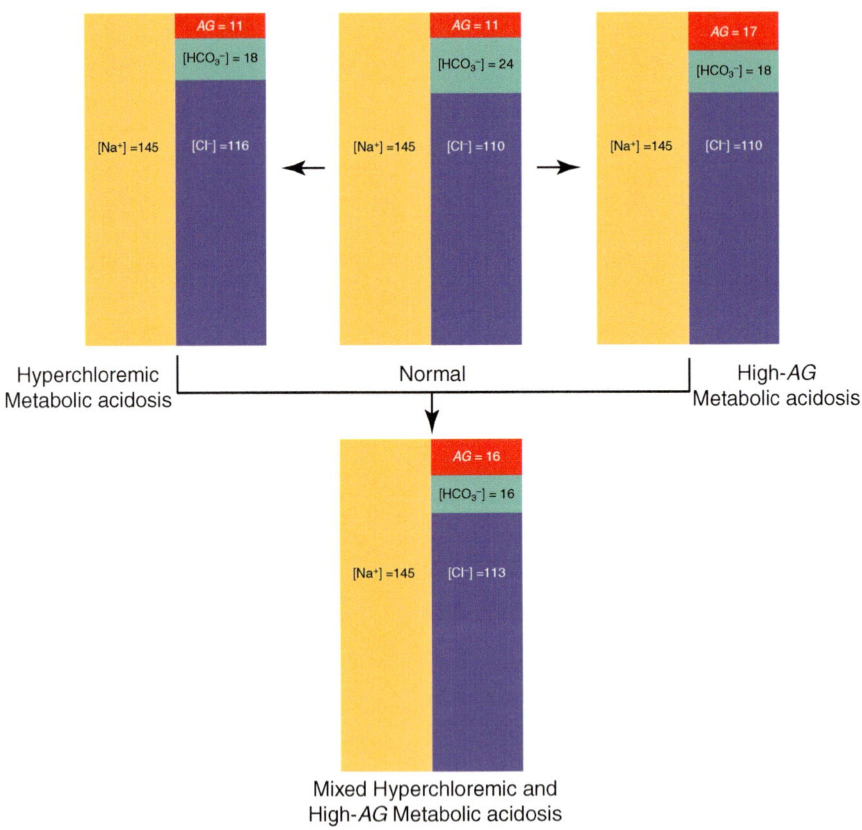

Fig. 8.1 Electrolyte composition in mixed hyperchloremic and high-*AG* metabolic acidosis

If $\Delta[Cl^-] = 0$, then:

$$\Delta\left[HCO_3^-\right] = \Delta AG$$

and we have a pure high-*AG* metabolic acidosis. On the other hand, if $\Delta AG = 0$, then:

$$\Delta\left[HCO_3^-\right] = \Delta\left[Cl^-\right]$$

and, a pure hyperchloremic (normal-*AG*) metabolic acidosis is present.

Finally, if neither ΔAG, nor $\Delta[Cl^-]$ equals zero, then a mixed hyperchloremic (normal-*AG*) and, high-*AG* metabolic acidosis should be present (Table 8.5).

Example A 16-year-old girl, a known case of insulin-dependent diabetes mellitus, was brought to the emergency room in a coma. According to her mother, the patient was well until 3 days before when she developed abdominal pain and then diarrhea. The day prior to admission she was unresponsive, and finally fell into coma. On physical examination, she was mildly dehydrated and feverish. Vital signs were measured as follows:

Temperature: 39.5 °C (orally), Pulse rate: 96/min (regular), Respiratory rate: 32/min (deep), Blood pressure: 100/70 mm Hg (supine position)

The pertinent laboratory exams were:

Arterial blood gas analysis:

$pCO_2 = 19$ mm Hg, $\left[HCO_3^-\right] = 8$ mEq/L, $pH = 7.246$, BE = −16.84 mEq/L

Serum chemistry:

$[Na^+] = 140$ mEq/L, $[K^+] = 5.1$ mEq/L, $[Cl^-] = 109$ mEq/L, Blood sugar = 510 mg/dL

Urinalysis: 2^+ Ketone, 3^+ Sugar

What is your diagnosis?

Solution: The very low *pH* and serum $\left[HCO_3^-\right]$ indicate a metabolic acidosis. A proportionate change in pCO_2 (Winter's formula) and a negative BE also support our diagnosis. Calculating the *AG*, we have:

Table 8.5 Electrolyte composition in mixed normal- and high-*AG* metabolic acidosis

Condition	*pH*	pCO_2	$\left[HCO_3^-\right]$	BE	$\Delta[Cl^-]$	ΔAG	Comment
High-*AG* Met. Ac.	↓	↓	↓	–	0	>0	$\Delta\left[HCO_3^-\right] = \Delta AG$
Mixed high-*AG* + Normal-*AG* Met. Ac.	↓	↓	↓	–	>0	>0	$\Delta\left[HCO_3^-\right] = \Delta AG + \Delta\left[Cl^-\right]$
Normal-*AG* Met. Ac.	↓	↓	↓	–	>0	0	$\Delta\left[HCO_3^-\right] = \Delta\left[Cl^-\right]$

Met. Metabolic, Ac. Acidosis

$$AG = [Na^+] - ([Cl^-] + [HCO_3^-])$$
$$= 140 - (109 + 8)$$
$$= 23\,mEq/L$$

Therefore:

$$\Delta AG = 23 - 12$$
$$= 11\,mEq/L$$

However, $\Delta[HCO_3^-]$ is 16 mEq/L (= 24–8) and exceeds ΔAG. Thus, as explained earlier, the patient has a mixed hyperchloremic and high-*AG* metabolic acidosis. The diarrhea causes the hyperchloremic component (loss of $[HCO_3^-]$ in exchange for Cl^-). The infection also causes fever and raises the body insulin demand and, finally, results in a diabetic ketoacidosis, the cause of the high-*AG* component (presence of ketoacids) [5]. The very high blood sugar concentration, 3^+ sugar, and 2^+ ketone in urine all support our diagnosis. Progression of this condition produces a more complex situation; fluid loss causes dehydration, which in turn results in tissue hypoperfusion and lactic acidosis, and metabolic alkalosis (kidneys reabsorb Na^+ and $[HCO_3^-]$ to preserve intravascular volume). Treatment in such a patient includes fluid and insulin therapy. Despite a high serum $[K^+]$, the total body potassium content is very low. Normalization of *pH* leads to severe hypokalemia. Therefore, potassium salts should also be given. Bicarbonate therapy is not necessary because during treatment the ketone bodies, themselves, change to bicarbonate.

The early stage of renal failure is associated with tubular damage, which causes a hyperchloremic acidosis. As kidney disease progresses, the glomerular failure results in a high-*AG* acidosis due to retention of phosphate, sulfate, and other anions. During this transitional state, we encounter a mixed hyperchloremic and high-*AG* metabolic acidosis.

8.3.3.2 Mixed High-*AG* Metabolic Acidosis $(\Delta AG = \Delta[HCO_3^-])$

When two high-*AG* acidosis coexist, e.g., lactic acidosis and ketoacidosis, the diagnosis is indistinguishable by the serum electrolyte composition alone, and only history and physical findings would suggest a mixed disorder [5, 6]. In these situations, measurement of specific substances such as plasma lactate or β-hydroxybutyrate may confirm the diagnosis. A variety of organic acids such as lactic and pyruvic acid in lactic acidosis, and β-hydroxybutyric and acetoacetic acid in ketoacidosis, may accumulate in high-*AG* acidosis. In diabetic ketoacidosis (a high-*AG* acidosis), the patient may develop lactic acidosis (another high-*AG* acidosis), due to impairment of lactic utilization, and this causes a mixed high-*AG* acidosis. Other conditions which may produce a mixed high-*AG* acidosis include glycogen storage disease, alcoholic acidosis, and certain intoxications (e.g., toxicity with methanol and ethylene glycol) [7].

8.3.3.3 Mixed Hyperchloremic Metabolic Acidosis ($\Delta AG = 0$)

Simultaneous occurrence of two hyperchloremic (normal-*AG*) acidosis results in a mixed hyperchloremic acidosis. As an example, a patient with RTA who developed diarrhea may develop a mixed hyperchloremic acidosis. In such cases, as in mixed high-*AG* acidosis, the only diagnostic clue may be found in history and physical examination.

8.3.4 Mixed Metabolic Acidosis and Metabolic Alkalosis

Occurrence of both metabolic acidosis and metabolic alkalosis results in little or no change in blood *pH* and serum $\left[HCO_3^-\right]$. Therefore, the respiratory drive will not change and pCO_2 remains normal (Table 8.6).

In a patient with high-*AG* metabolic acidosis, the decrement in plasma $\left[HCO_3^-\right]$ is just equal to the increase in the *AG* $\left(\Delta AG = \Delta\left[HCO_3^-\right]\right)$. When a metabolic alkalosis is superimposed on a high-*AG* metabolic acidosis (e.g., nasogastric suction in a patient with diabetic ketoacidosis, alkali therapy in a uremic patient, or severe vomiting and dehydration) serum $\left[HCO_3^-\right]$ and *pH* return toward normal, but the *AG* remains high. Therefore, failure of the serum $\left[HCO_3^-\right]$ to fall by an amount equal to the increase in *AG* $\left(\Delta AG > \Delta\left[HCO_3^-\right]\right)$ is the only laboratory clue to the presence of a mixed high-*AG* metabolic acidosis and metabolic alkalosis. On the other hand, when a hyperchloremic (normal-*AG*) metabolic acidosis coexists with a metabolic alkalosis (e.g., a patient with gastroenteritis who develops diarrhea and vomiting), all laboratory data may be normal (*pH*, pCO_2, $\left[HCO_3^-\right]$, and *AG*). In this condition (as in mixed high-*AG* acidosis and mixed hyperchloremic metabolic acidosis), the diagnosis may be built only upon the history and physical examination.

Table 8.6 Blood gas values in mixed metabolic acidosis and metabolic alkalosis

Condition	*pH*	pCO_2	$\left[HCO_3^-\right]$	BE	Comment
Met. Ac.	↓	↓	↓	–	$pCO_2 = 1.5\left[HCO_3^-\right] + 8 \pm 2$ > 10mm Hg
Mixed Met. Ac. + Met. Al.	?	?	?	?	The only diagnostic clue may be found in *AG*, history, and physical examination
Met. Al.	↑	↑	↑	+	$\Delta pCO_2 = (0.4 \text{ to } 0.9)\Delta\left[HCO_3^-\right]$ or $pCO_2 = 0.5\left[HCO_3^-\right] + 28 \pm 4$ < 55mm Hg

Met. Metabolic, Ac. Acidosis, Al. Alkalosis, ? Unpredictable—low, normal, or high

8.3.5 Mixed Metabolic Alkalosis and Respiratory Acidosis; Mixed Metabolic and Respiratory Alkalosis

A primary increase in serum $\left[HCO_3^-\right]$ causes a metabolic alkalosis, which is not only frequently seen as a pure disorder, but may also commonly occur concomitantly with other acid-base disturbances. This pathologic process (metabolic alkalosis) is followed by a compensatory depression of the respiratory center and, finally, CO_2 retention.

As we saw earlier (Chapter 6), the predicted value for the pCO_2 after respiratory compensation can be calculated by either of the following equations:

$$\Delta pCO_2 = (0.4 \text{ to } 0.9)\Delta\left[HCO_3^-\right]$$

$$pCO_2 = 0.5\left[HCO_3^-\right] + 28 \pm 4$$

If the patient's pCO_2 is significantly higher than the predicted value, then a mixed metabolic alkalosis and respiratory acidosis should coexist (Table 8.7). On the other hand, a pCO_2 markedly lower than that predicted means the presence of a mixed metabolic and respiratory alkalosis (Table 8.8).

Example A 40-year-old man with liver cirrhosis and refractory edema was admitted to the hospital for liver transplantation. Everything went well until a day before the operation, when he developed a high-grade fever and a productive cough. Chest roentgenography revealed bilateral pleural effusion and diffuse interstitial infiltration. Pertinent laboratory exams were as follows:

pCO_2 = 53 mm Hg, $\left[HCO_3^-\right]$ = 34 mEq/L, pH = 7.429, BE = 9.24 mEq/L
Explain the above abnormal values.

Table 8.7 Blood gas in mixed metabolic alkalosis and respiratory acidosis

Condition	*pH*	pCO_2	$\left[HCO_3^-\right]$	BE	Comment
Met. Al.	↑	↑	↑	+	$\Delta pCO_2 = (0.4 \text{ to } 0.9)\Delta\left[HCO_3^-\right]$ or $pCO_2 = 0.5\left[HCO_3^-\right] + 28 \pm 4$ < 55 mm Hg
Mixed Met. Al. + R. Ac.	?	↑↑	↑↑	+	$pCO_2 >$ Predicted value or $\left[HCO_3^-\right] >$ Predicted value
R. Ac.	↓	↑	↑	+	$\Delta\left[HCO_3^-\right]_{Acute} = 0.1\,\Delta pCO_2 \pm 2$ $\left[HCO_3^-\right]_{Acute} < 30$ mm Hg $\Delta\left[HCO_3^-\right]_{Chronic} = 0.4\,\Delta pCO_2 \pm 2$ $\left[HCO_3^-\right]_{Acute} < 45$ mm Hg

Met. Metabolic, R. Respiratory, Ac. Acidosis, Al. Alkalosis, ? Unpredictable—low, normal, or high

Table 8.8 Blood gas values in mixed metabolic and respiratory alkalosis

Condition	*pH*	pCO_2	$\left[HCO_3^-\right]$	BE	Comment
Met. Al.	↑	↑	↑	+	$\Delta pCO_2 = (0.4 \text{ to } 0.9)\Delta\left[HCO_3^-\right]$ or $pCO_2 = 0.5\left[HCO_3^-\right] + 28 \pm 4$ < 55 mm Hg
Mixed Met. Al. + R. Al.	↑↑	?	?	?	$pCO_2 <$ Predicted value or $\left[HCO_3^-\right] >$ Predicted value
R. Al.	↑	↓	↓	−	$\Delta\left[HCO_3^-\right]_{Acute} = 0.2\,\Delta pCO_2 \pm 2$ $\left[HCO_3^-\right]_{Acute} > 18$ mm Hg $\Delta\left[HCO_3^-\right]_{Chronic} = 0.5\,\Delta pCO_2 \pm 2$ $\left[HCO_3^-\right]_{Acute} > 12$ mm Hg

Met. Metabolic, R. Respiratory, Al. Alkalosis, ? Unpredictable—low, normal, or high

Solution: Although *pH* is within normal range, high serum $\left[HCO_3^-\right]$, pCO_2, and BE indicate the presence of a problem. Regarding high serum $\left[HCO_3^-\right]$ and positive BE, the condition is in favor of a metabolic alkalosis, and hypercapnia and positive BE, suggest a respiratory acidosis. Using Eq. (7.4), we have:

$$\begin{aligned}\Delta pCO_2 &= (0.4 \text{ to } 0.9)\Delta\left[HCO_3^-\right]\\ &= (0.4 \text{ to } 0.9)\times(34-24)\\ &= (0.4 \text{ to } 0.9)\times 10\\ &= 4 \text{ to } 9 \text{ mm Hg}\end{aligned}$$

then:

$$\begin{aligned}pCO_2 &= 40 + (4 \text{ to } 9)\\ &= 44 \text{ to } 49 \text{ mm Hg}\end{aligned}$$

Equation (7.5) results in an almost similar expected values:

$$\begin{aligned}pCO_2 &= 0.5\left[HCO_3^-\right] + 28 \pm 4\\ &= 0.5\times 34 + 28 \pm 4\\ &= 45 \pm 4 \text{ mm Hg}\end{aligned}$$

The measured pCO_2 (53 mm Hg) is significantly higher than the maximum limit of the expected value (49 mm Hg), indicating a coexistent respiratory acidosis.

The patient had a mixed metabolic alkalosis and respiratory acidosis. The metabolic alkalosis can be explained by the use of multiple diuretics due to the refractory edema, and the superimposed respiratory component is interpreted to be due to the lung disease. Since there was not enough time for the kidneys to compensate this respiratory disturbance (only 1 day), it is better to state that our patient had a mixed metabolic alkalosis and acute (or partially compensated) respiratory acidosis. Do not forget that even after full compensation of a metabolic alkalosis, the pCO_2 rarely exceeds 55 mm Hg, and a measured pCO_2 *higher than 55 mm Hg per se suggests the presence of a respiratory acidosis* (Tables 8.1 and 8.7).

All the above occur if the primary disturbance is a metabolic alkalosis. If the primary disorder is assumed to be a respiratory acidosis, the serum $\left[HCO_3^-\right]$ in the acute and chronic phase of compensation can be obtained by (see Eqs. (6.1), (6.2) below):

$$\left.\begin{array}{r}\text{Acute phase: } \Delta\left[HCO_3^-\right] = 0.1\ \Delta pCO_2 \pm 2 \\ \text{Chronic phase: } \Delta\left[HCO_3^-\right] = 0.4\ \Delta pCO_2 \pm 2\end{array}\right\}$$

A serum $\left[HCO_3^-\right]$ significantly higher than these predicted values implies the coexistence of a metabolic alkalosis, whereas a plasma $\left[HCO_3^-\right]$ significantly lower than the calculated values indicates a mixed respiratory and metabolic acidosis. The type of the metabolic component (i.e., hyperchloremic or high-*AG*) can be easily identified by the examination of serum electrolytes and the *AG*.

Example A 32-year-old man, who was injured in a car accident, was admitted to the ICU. On admission, he was in deep coma. An endotracheal tube was inserted and mechanical ventilatory assist was started. Also, a urinary catheter and a nasogastric tube attached to an intermittent suction were inserted. Five hours later, his arterial blood gas analysis revealed:

$pCO_2 = 27$ mm Hg, $\left[HCO_3^-\right] = 26$ mEq/L, $pH = 7.605$, BE = 6.39 mEq/L.

Explain the blood gas values.

Solution: The presented alkalemia with associated hypocapnia show a respiratory alkalosis. Regarding the history, the problem should be acute, thus, Eq. (6.3) should be used:

$$\begin{aligned}\Delta\left[HCO_3^-\right] &= 0.2\ \Delta pCO_2 \pm 2 \\ &= 0.2 \times 13 \pm 2 \\ &= 2.6 \pm 2\ \text{mEq / L}\end{aligned}$$

As a result, if the patient has an acute respiratory alkalosis, the serum $\left[HCO_3^-\right]$ should range from 19.4 to 23.4 (= 24–2.6 ± 2) mEq/L. Nevertheless, the measured plasma $\left[HCO_3^-\right]$ significantly exceeds the expected value, reflecting the presence of a metabolic alkalosis. Therefore, the diagnosis is mixed acute respiratory alkalosis (due to hyperventilation) and metabolic alkalosis (due to nasogastric suction). However, we may think that there is another way of approach, that is to say that regarding alkalemia with a high serum $\left[HCO_3^-\right]$ and a positive BE, a metabolic alkalosis is suggested. Using Eq. (7.4), then:

$$\begin{aligned}\Delta pCO_2 &= (0.4 \text{ to } 0.9)\Delta\left[HCO_3^-\right]\\ &= (0.4 \text{ to } 0.9)\times(26-24)\\ &= (0.4 \text{ to } 0.9)\times 2\\ &= 0.8 \text{ to } 1.8 \text{ mm Hg}\end{aligned}$$

Then:

$$\begin{aligned}pCO_2 &= 40+(0.8 \text{ to } 1.8)\\ &= 40.8 \text{ to } 41.8 \text{ mm Hg}\end{aligned}$$

The measured pCO_2 (27 mm Hg) is significantly lower than the expected value (40.8 mm Hg). Thus, the patient also has a respiratory alkalosis. Correct?

Wrong! The observed difference in pCO_2 arises for two reasons: (1) There is a ventilator which controls the patient's respiratory rate and tidal volume; thus, *there could be no respiratory compensation*; and (2) even if there was no ventilator at all, the compensation for a metabolic alkalosis needs at least 12–24 h (Table 8.1) to be completed. During this period, the pCO_2 rises and it is certainly less than what we may find from Eq. (7.4) or (7.5) (which is only true after full compensation). Thereby, using Eqs. (7.4) and (7.5) before a full compensation leads to a misdiagnosis of a mixed condition; respiratory alkalosis superimposed a metabolic alkalosis. Therefore, the second approach is incomplete; that is, we can only state that although the patient has a metabolic alkalosis, it cannot be clear as to whether or not he has a respiratory alkalosis. We should rely on our first diagnosis; mixed acute respiratory alkalosis and metabolic alkalosis, even though it is the same as the second one, yet derived from the right way. H_2 blocking agents, such as cimetidine (Tagamet) suppress gastric acid secretion, thus relieving the metabolic component of acid-base in this patient. Moreover, they help in preventing peptic ulcer (stress ulcer), which is not uncommon in such patients.

As a general rule, a normal or near-normal blood *pH*, with a very abnormal plasma $\left[HCO_3^-\right]$ and pCO_2, should be explained as a mixed metabolic and respiratory disorder.

Severe alkalemia has multiple adverse effects on the central nervous system (CNS) and cardiovascular system (CVS); its treatment is therefore, mandatory. If the patient is under ventilator, pCO_2 should be increased by lowering the ventilation (thus, producing a respiratory acidosis); otherwise, treatment is difficult and the underlying cause of alkalemia must be corrected. The treatment, as before, should be directed at removal of the underlying disorder. As an example, volume, chloride, and potassium deficit should be corrected and treatment of the underlying cause of hyperventilation (e.g., sepsis, pain, and trauma) should be started.

8.3.6 Mixed Acute and Chronic Respiratory Acidosis or Alkalosis

In chronic respiratory acidosis (e.g., a patient with COPD), the pCO_2 is high, and metabolic compensation causes an appropriate increase in serum $\left[HCO_3^-\right]$. If a chronic respiratory acidosis is complicated by an acute respiratory acidosis (e.g., pneumonia in a patient with COPD), the blood gas analysis reveals a very high pCO_2, and an elevated serum $\left[HCO_3^-\right]$ which is lower than the predicted value for a pure compensated chronic respiratory acidosis (Eq. (6.2)). Thus, the diagnosis may be (1) a chronic respiratory acidosis which is superimposed by either a metabolic or an acute respiratory acidosis, or (2) an acute respiratory acidosis superimposed by a metabolic alkalosis. Then, the only diagnostic clue may be found in history and physical examination.

Treatment of this condition should be directed at the treatment of the underlying superimposing problem and the provision of some ventilatory support.

Example Which of these conditions are consistent with the following blood gas values?

$pCO_2 = 58$ mm Hg, $\left[HCO_3^-\right] = 28.6$ mEq/L, $pH = 7.314$, BE = 1.88 mEq/L

(a) A patient with chronic bronchitis develops persistent diarrhea.
(b) A 55-year-old woman with chronic emphysema complains of fever and increased sputum production. The chest X-ray is consistent with pneumonia.
(c) A 2-year-old boy with foreign body aspiration who develops multiple episodes of vomiting.
(d) All of the above
(e) None of the above

Solution: Regarding acidemia and hypercapnia, the diagnosis is a respiratory acidosis. BE although positive, is within normal limits (−2 to +2 mEq/L), indicating that, if the problem is a simple acid-base disorder, there has been no time for compensation, and thus it must be an acute respiratory acidosis. Using Eq. (6.1) (acute phase), we have:

$$\begin{aligned}\Delta\left[HCO_3^-\right] &= 0.1\,\Delta pCO_2 \pm 2\\ &= 0.1\times(58-40)\pm 2\\ &= 0.1\times 18\pm 2\\ &= 1.8\pm 2\ \text{mEq / L}\end{aligned}$$

Therefore, the expected serum $\left[HCO_3^-\right]$ is from 23.8 to 27.8 mEq/L. However, the measured plasma $\left[HCO_3^-\right]$ exceeds the upper limit of this range, thus the diagnosis is a metabolic alkalosis over an acute respiratory acidosis. Therefore, answer "c" is correct. The foreign body causes an acute respiratory acidosis, and the reflex vomiting superimposes a metabolic alkalosis. Nevertheless, as we found, the problem is not a simple acid-base disorder but a mixed one; therefore, we cannot rely on BE to state that the original disturbance is an acute process; as, in mixed disorders, the components may cancel out their effects on BE and cause a normal value. Therefore, considering the acidemia and hypercapnia, the original disorder may be a chronic respiratory acidosis. Employing Eq. (6.2) (chronic phase), we have:

$$\Delta\left[HCO_3^-\right] = 0.4\ \Delta pCO_2 \pm 2$$
$$= 0.4 \times (58 - 40) \pm 2$$
$$= 0.4 \times 18 \pm 2$$
$$= 7.2 \pm 2\,\text{mEq / L}$$

Therefore, the expected serum $\left[HCO_3^-\right]$ is from 29.2 to 33.2 mEq/L. However, here the measured plasma $\left[HCO_3^-\right]$ (28.6 mEq/L) is significantly lower than that expected. Thus, the diagnosis should be a metabolic acidosis over a chronic respiratory acidosis; that is, the answer "a" is correct. The chronic bronchitis is the cause of chronic respiratory acidosis, and the diarrhea causes the superimposed metabolic acidosis. As it was found, the measured serum $\left[HCO_3^-\right]$ (28.6 mEq/L) is neither appropriate for an acute respiratory acidosis, nor is compatible with a chronic one, but is something intermediary, indicating that the problem may be a combination of a chronic and acute respiratory acidosis. As a result, answer "b" may also be another correct choice. The chronic emphysema causes a chronic respiratory acidosis and the pneumonia imposes an acute respiratory acidosis over it. Therefore, the answer should be "d" (all of the above). This is why we emphasize history and physical examination.

Chronic respiratory alkalosis is characterized by a low pCO_2 and a modest decrease in plasma $\left[HCO_3^-\right]$. It may be accompanied by an acute respiratory alkalosis, for example, secondary to anxiety. In such cases, the pCO_2 is usually very low, and the serum $\left[HCO_3^-\right]$ is decreased; however, it is higher than the predicted value for a pure compensated chronic respiratory alkalosis (Eq. (6.4)). In such conditions, mixed chronic respiratory and metabolic alkalosis, and mixed acute respiratory alkalosis and metabolic acidosis should be ruled out by re-evaluating the history and physical findings.

Example Which of these conditions are consistent with the following blood gas values?

$pCO_2 = 24$ mm Hg, $\left[HCO_3^-\right] = 18.5$ mEq/L, $pH = 7.508$, BE = −1.65 mEq/L

(a) A 26-year-old woman with Gram-negative sepsis who has ileus. A nasogastric tube is inserted and attached to an intermittent suction.
(b) A patient with pulmonary emboli who develops heart failure
(c) A 25-year-old comatose patient under ventilator
(d) All of the above
(e) None of the above

Solution: Considering the alkalemia and hypocapnia, the diagnosis should be a respiratory alkalosis. However, although BE is negative it is within normal range (−2 to +2 mEq/L); therefore, if the problem is a simple (not mixed) disorder it should be an acute one. Employing Eq. (6.3) (acute phase), we have:

$$\begin{aligned}\Delta\left[HCO_3^-\right] &= 0.2\ \Delta pCO_2 \pm 2\\ &= 0.2\times(40-24)\pm 2\\ &= 0.2\times 16\pm 2\\ &= 3.2\pm 2\,\text{mEq/L}\end{aligned}$$

Therefore, the expected serum $\left[HCO_3^-\right]$ is from 18.8 to 22.8 mEq/L. Nevertheless, the measured plasma $\left[HCO_3^-\right]$ (18.5 mEq/L) is lower than that expected. Thereby, the diagnosis should be a mixed metabolic acidosis over an acute respiratory alkalosis. Thus, answer "b" is correct; pulmonary emboli causes the acute respiratory alkalosis and the heart failure produces hypotension, tissue hypoperfusion, and the resultant metabolic acidosis (lactic acidosis). However, as it was found, the disorder is not simple but a mixed acid-base disorder. Thus, we cannot rely on BE to state that the original problem is an acute process as in mixed conditions the components may oppose their effects on BE and cause a normal value. Therefore, considering the alkalemia and hypocapnia, the original disorder may be a chronic respiratory alkalosis. Employing Eq. (6.4) (chronic phase), we have:

$$\begin{aligned}\Delta\left[HCO_3^-\right] &= 0.5\ \Delta pCO_2 \pm 2\\ &= 0.5\times(40-24)\pm 2\\ &= 0.5\times 16\pm 2\\ &= 8\pm 2\ \text{mEq/L}\end{aligned}$$

Thus, the expected serum $\left[HCO_3^-\right]$ is from 14 to 18 mEq/L, but here the measured plasma $\left[HCO_3^-\right]$ (18.5 mEq/L) exceeds the upper limit of this range. Therefore, the diagnosis should be a metabolic alkalosis over a chronic respiratory alkalosis. That is, the answer "a" is correct. Gram-negative sepsis causes a chronic respiratory alkalosis, and nasogastric suction imposes a metabolic alkalosis over it. As it was found, the measured serum $\left[HCO_3^-\right]$ (18.5 mEq/L) is neither appropriate for an acute respiratory alkalosis, nor consistent with a chronic one, but is something midway, indicating that the problem may be a combination of a chronic and acute respiratory alkalosis. As a result, answer "c" may also be another correct choice. A patient under ventilator may have any form of respiratory acid-base disorders (because his respiration is actually in your hand, and you may do anything you wish). Therefore, the answer should be "d" (all of the above). This is why we emphasize on history and physical examination.

8.3.7 Triple Acid-Base Disorders

When three primary acid-base disturbances occur simultaneously, a triple acid-base disorder is present. In such situations, history and physical examination are again the most important parts of the diagnosis.

Example A 57-year-old man who had had asthma for 40 years was admitted to the emergency room because of sudden dyspnea and squeezing chest pain following severe exertion. On arrival, he was cyanotic; auscultation of the lung revealed bilateral basilar wet rales. His blood pressure was 85/50 mm Hg (supine position). It was inferred that he had had a myocardial infarction; it was later confirmed. The arterial blood gas analysis initially was reported as:

$pCO_2 = 56$ mm Hg, $\left[HCO_3^-\right] = 29$ mEq/L, $pH = 7.365$, BE = 4.96 mEq/L

However, 5 h later, the second one revealed:

$pCO_2 = 67$ mm Hg, $\left[HCO_3^-\right] = 22$ mEq/L, $pH = 7.157$, BE = −6.89 mEq/L

At the same time, the serum chemistry was:

$[Na^+] = 139$ mEq/L, $[K^+] = 5.1$ mEq/L, $[Cl^-] = 92$ mEq/L

Explain the acid-base condition.

Solution: The initial values of blood gas show hypercapnia and a mild acidemia. The bicarbonate level is consistent with a chronic respiratory acidosis (Eq. (6.2)):

$$\begin{aligned}\Delta\left[HCO_3^-\right] &= 0.4\ \Delta pCO_2 \pm 2\\ &= 0.4\times(56-40)\pm 2\\ &= 0.4\times 16\pm 2 = 0.4\times 16\pm 2\\ &= 6.4\pm 2\ \text{mEq / L}\end{aligned}$$

This chronic respiratory acidosis is because of the chronic lung disease in our patient. In the second blood gas analysis, however, we have an acute rise in pCO_2, and plasma $\left[HCO_3^-\right]$ is decreased significantly. Besides, the BE from a positive value (4.96 mEq/L), which in this case indicates a chronic respiratory acidosis, falls to a negative value (−6.89 mEq/L). Since there is no reason for having a respiratory alkalosis, this fall in BE declares a metabolic acidosis (a negative BE means either a compensated respiratory alkalosis or a metabolic acidosis). Moreover, calculating the *AG* (Eq. (5.2)) reveals:

$$\begin{aligned}AG &= \left[Na^+\right]-\left(\left[Cl^-\right]+\left[HCO_3^-\right]\right)\\ &= 139-(92+22)\\ &= 25\ \text{mEq / L}\end{aligned}$$

A value significantly higher than the normal value (12 ± 2 mEq/L). The presence of bilateral basilar wet rales is indicative for pulmonary edema. The myocardial infarction caused heart failure and pulmonary edema. The resultant pulmonary edema, in turn, induced an acute rise in pCO_2 and led to acute respiratory acidosis, which was superimposed on the primary chronic respiratory acidosis. On the other hand, hypotension, which was the consequence of low cardiac output, caused tissue hypoperfusion and finally lactic acidosis (high *AG*, and decreased serum $\left[HCO_3^-\right]$ and BE). Therefore, the diagnosis is a triple acid-base disturbance—mixed chronic respiratory acidosis, acute respiratory acidosis, and high-*AG* metabolic acidosis.

The treatment should include ventilatory assist and sufficient oxygenation to treat the acute respiratory acidosis and circulatory support to alleviate the metabolic component.

In a patient with metabolic acidosis and alkalosis, the net effect of the opposing metabolic disturbances determines the final serum $\left[HCO_3^-\right]$ and *pH*. Depending on the resultant metabolic state, the proper respiratory compensation occurs. If the measured pCO_2 exceeds the predicted pCO_2, then a mixed metabolic alkalosis, metabolic acidosis, and respiratory acidosis is the diagnosis. On the other hand, if the measured pCO_2 is lower than the predicted pCO_2, then a mixed metabolic alkalosis, metabolic acidosis, and respiratory alkalosis should be considered.

Finally, it is worth remembering that the components of a mixed condition exert either additive or opposing effects on each other. It is the algebraic sum of these influences that determines the final blood *pH* and electrolyte composition.

8.4 Things to Remember

The mixed acid-base conditions are commonly seen in the clinical practice. Hence, their diagnosis and treatment are very important. Any simple (non-mixed) acid-base derangement, either respiratory or metabolic, shows its own characteristic features. As an example, in acute respiratory acidosis the change in serum $\left[HCO_3^-\right]$ is about 1 mEq/L for each 10 mm Hg raise in arterial pCO_2. Any significant deviation from this expected behavior indicates a mixed disorder. For example, in a patient expected to have an acute respiratory acidosis, a measured $\left[HCO_3^-\right]$ higher than the expected value reveals the coexistence of a metabolic alkalosis. To be able to have a good judgment in such conditions, the expected behavior of each simple acid-base disturbance should be well known, and this is what you can find in Table 8.1. Thus:

1. Look at the blood *pH*.
2. Find the primary disturbance based on history, physical examination, arterial pCO_2, serum $\left[HCO_3^-\right]$, and BE.
3. Calculate the expected range of compensation.
4. If the level of compensation is within the expected range, your patient has a simple acid-base problem.
5. Otherwise, the patient has a mixed acid-base disturbance.
6. Subsequently find the other acid-base disturbance(s) based on serum chemistry and the *AG*.
7. Start the proper treatment, if it is necessary.

A normal *pH* does not rule out a mixed problem. In such cases, proper analysis of history, physical examination, and serum chemistry is essential for framing the final diagnosis.

At any time, do not forget that the history and physical examination are your most important guides, and you should never underestimate them.

References

1. Adams LG, Polzin DJ. Mixed acid-base disorders. Vet Clin North Am Small Anim Pract. 1989;19(2):307–26. https://doi.org/10.1016/s0195-5616(89)50032-9.
2. Narins RG, Emmett M. Simple and mixed acid-base disorders: a practical approach. Medicine (Baltimore). 1980;59(3):161–87. https://doi.org/10.1097/00005792-198005000-00001.
3. Palmer BF, Clegg DJ. Salicylate toxicity. N Engl J Med. 2020;382(26):2544–55. https://doi.org/10.1056/NEJMra2010852.
4. Mandell I. Serum anion gap in metabolic acidosis. Neonatal Netw. 2009;28(4):252–4; quiz 5-8. https://doi.org/10.1891/0730-0832.28.4.252.
5. Trachtenbarg DE. Diabetic ketoacidosis. Am Fam Physician. 2005;71(9):1705–14.
6. Kraut JA, Madias NE. Lactic acidosis. N Engl J Med. 2014;371(24):2309–19. https://doi.org/10.1056/NEJMra1309483.
7. Brubaker RH, Vashisht R, Meseeha M. High anion gap metabolic acidosis. Treasure Island, FL: StatPearls; 2020.

Arterial Blood Gas

9

9.1 Hypoxia and Its Causes

Adequate tissue oxygenation and CO_2 elimination depend on pulmonary ventilation and perfusion, blood-gas exchange, and tissue perfusion [1, 2]. Hypoxia (decreased oxygen supply to tissues, despite sufficient tissue perfusion) is due to the following reasons [3]:

9.1.1 Ventilation-Perfusion ($\dot{V}/\dot{Q}$) Mismatch

$\dot{V}/\dot{Q}$ mismatch results from either the continued ventilation of alveoli which are poorly perfused (e.g., pulmonary emboli) (Fig. 9.1), or perfusion of underventilated alveoli (e.g., foreign body aspiration, atelectasis, excessive airway secretions, pulmonary edema, or lung cancer) (Fig. 9.1).

Blood perfusing these underventilated alveoli does not become oxygenated completely; thus, it has a lower oxygen tension and decreases the total intermixed left atrial blood pO_2. If the $\dot{V}/\dot{Q}$ mismatch is large enough, it may diminish the average pO_2, even to a subnormal value.

9.1.2 Blood Shunt

The extreme form of $\dot{V}/\dot{Q}$ mismatch is blood shunt, in which the amount of unoxygenated blood is high enough to cause a significant reduction in p_aO_2 (Fig. 9.2). In the presence of a shunt, a large portion of blood either perfuses the unventilated alveoli or passes directly from the right side to the left side of the heart via a congenital defect. The latter condition is usually called cyanotic heart disease [4].

In the case of $\dot{V}/\dot{Q}$ mismatch, p_aO_2 may be raised by increasing the inspired oxygen concentration (f_iO_2), whereas augmentation of f_iO_2 has little or no effect on

F. Habibzadeh et al., *Pathophysiologic Basis of Acid-Base Disorders*,
https://doi.org/10.1007/978-981-16-0526-0_9

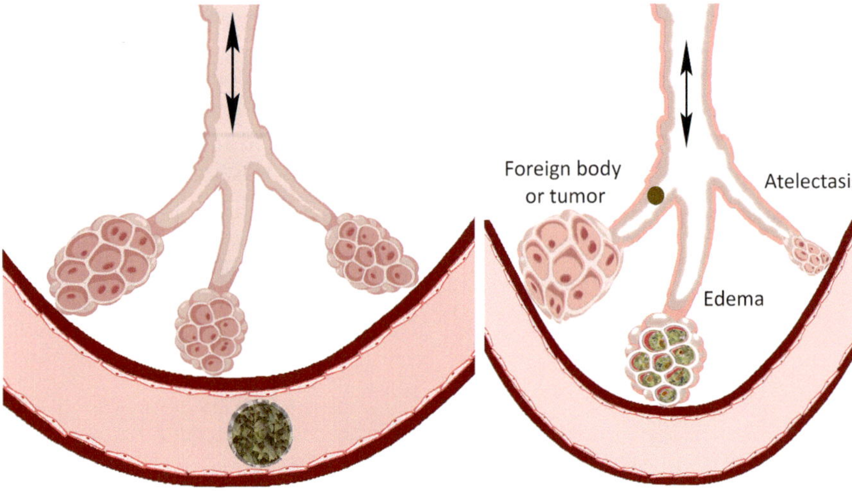

Fig. 9.1 Some causes of ventilation/perfusion mismatch: (left panel) ventilation of poorly perfused alveoli, and (right panel) perfusion of underventilated alveoli

Fig. 9.2 Blood shunt is a cause of hypoxia

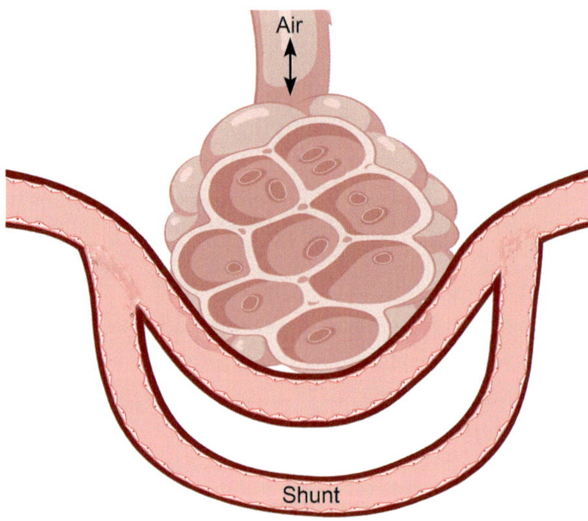

the shunt. Therefore, a simple clinical method to determine the presence of a shunt and also measure its percentage (percentage of cardiac output which is involved) is to measure p_aO_2 before and after 20 min of breathing 100% oxygen. This maneuver causes the alveolar pO_2 of even the most underventilated alveoli to increase to 100 mm Hg, thus eliminating any alveolar-arterial pO_2 difference due to $\dot{V}/\dot{Q}$ mismatch. In the presence of shunt, the p_aO_2 has little or no increase, whereas it reaches a normal value in the case of $\dot{V}/\dot{Q}$ mismatch.

Alveolar-arterial pO_2 difference ($p_{(A\text{-}a)}O_2$) is defined as [2]:

$$p_{(A\text{-}a)}O_2 = p_AO_2 - p_aO_2$$

In a normal young person, $p_{(A-a)}O_2$ averages 8 mm Hg; it linearly increases with age. As an example, the normal value for $p_{(A-a)}O_2$ is up to 17 mm Hg in a 75-year-old man because of changes in the permeability of the alveolar membrane which results in a decreased p_aO_2, without any change in p_AO_2. In general, in patients breathing room-air this difference should not exceed 10 mm Hg; with an f_iO_2 high enough to provide a p_AO_2 of 200 mm Hg or more, the $p_{(A-a)}O_2$ should not be more than 40 mm Hg.

There are some normally presented anatomic shunts of blood from the systemic veins (unoxygenated) into the pulmonary venous blood (oxygenated); examples are Thebesian veins of the left ventricle and bronchial vein. There are also some regions with imbalanced $\dot{V}/\dot{Q}$. These two normally existing processes are responsible for the reduced intermixed blood pO_2 and an alveolar-arterial O_2 pressure difference.

Any increase in $p_{(A-a)}O_2$ suggests either excess anatomic shunt of blood through the lung or other shunts elsewhere. Defect in diffusion and oxygen transport across the alveolar-capillary barrier is also a major cause of elevated $p_{(A-a)}O_2$ (e.g., when the distance between the alveoli and pulmonary capillaries is increased by fibrous tissue or inflammatory exudate).

9.1.3 Hypoventilation

Because of hypoventilation (e.g., opium poisoning) insufficient oxygen is provided to the alveoli and the p_aO_2 drops. The only necessary therapeutic measure in such conditions is to improve ventilation. As there is no problem in the carriage of oxygen from alveoli to blood, the $p_{(A-a)}O_2$ is within normal range.

9.1.4 Thickening of Blood-Gas Interface

The blood-gas barrier thickness is less than 0.5 μm. In certain disease conditions (e.g., pulmonary edema, asbestosis), the thickness of the blood-gas interface (the distance between the alveoli and pulmonary capillaries) may be increased by edema, fluid, fibrous tissue, and the presence of inflammatory cells. This disturbs gas diffusion and may lead to hypoxemia (Fig. 9.3).

In hypoxic states which are associated with hypercapnia, a normal $p_{(A-a)}O_2$ is diagnostic for alveolar hypoventilation, whereas an abnormally high $p_{(A-a)}O_2$ suggests that a lung disease (e.g., a diffusion defect) is also present. A negative or near--zero $p_{(A-a)}O_2$ reflects a laboratory or calculation error in all circumstances.

Serial values of $p_{(A-a)}O_2$ are useful for follow-up of a progressive lung disease; they can be employed as a guide for weaning from mechanical ventilation. Some causes of increased $p_{(A-a)}O_2$ are given in Table 9.1.

9.2 Oxyhemoglobin Dissociation Curve

In chapter 4, the significant sigmoid shape of oxyhemoglobin dissociation curve and its physiologic consequences were thoroughly explained (Fig. 9.4). Here, we show you some key points which have clinical significance, so you can find the place of your patient on the curve, and reasonably determine his oxygenation status.

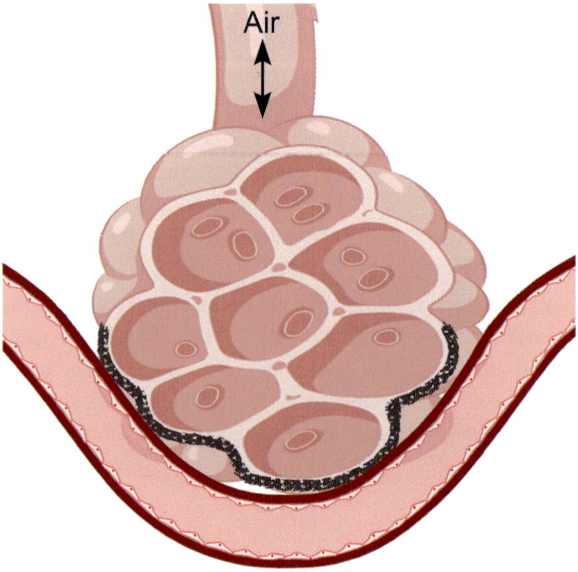

Fig. 9.3 Thickening of blood-gas barrier is a cause of hypoxia

Table 9.1 Some causes of increased $p_{(A-a)}O_2$

Post-traumatic pulmonary insufficiency
Sepsis
Aspiration of gastric contents
Respiratory burns/smoke inhalation
Inhalation of toxic chemicals
Chlorine
Mustard gas
Viral pneumonia
Left-to-right blood shunts
Fat embolism
Uremia
Pancreatitis
Oxygen toxicity
Pulmonary edema
Neurogenic
Altitude-induced

Referring to this Figure, which is redrawn from chapter 4, you can distinguish these points easily. If $HbO_2\%$ represents hemoglobin oxygen saturation, these key points are:

1. *The point with pO_2 of 20 mm Hg and $HbO_2\%$ of 35%:* this point indicates a life-threatening hypoxemia. At this point, the patient has a very poor oxygenation state, and sufficient oxygen should be given promptly.

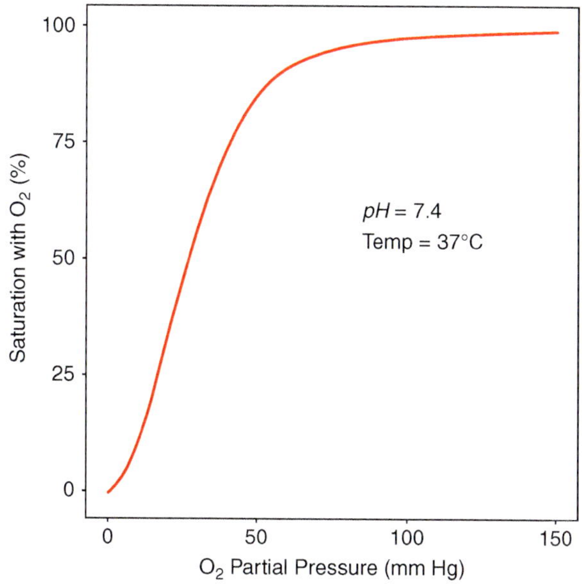

Fig. 9.4 Oxyhemoglobin dissociation curve

2. *The point with pO_2 of 40 mm Hg and $HbO_2\%$ of 75%:* this is the level at which cyanosis is clearly detectable, provided blood hemoglobin concentration is normal.
3. *The point with pO_2 of 60 mm Hg and $HbO_2\%$ of 90%:* this is the shoulder of the oxyhemoglobin dissociation curve. Below this point, the curve is steep. As it was explained earlier (Chapter 4), this region has a very important physiologic role. In this portion of the curve, a slight change in pO_2 causes a great change in $HbO_2\%$, thus facilitating tissue oxygenation (see Chapter 4).
4. *The point with pO_2 of 80 mm Hg and $HbO_2\%$ of 95%:* these are the normal arterial values for an elderly individual.
5. *The point with pO_2 of 100 mm Hg and $HbO_2\%$ of 97%:* these are the normal arterial values for a young person.

Example A 20-year-old woman with sedative overdose was brought to the emergency room. On admission, the patient was in coma; her pupils were bilaterally pinpoint size; and her respiratory rate was 10 breaths per minute. The arterial blood gas analysis at the same time revealed:

$pCO_2 = 61$ mm Hg, $\left[HCO_3^-\right] = 26.7$ mEq/L, $pH = 7.263$, BE = −0.79 mEq/L, $pO_2 = 65$ mm Hg. If the patient has no fever and breathes the ambient air under a barometric pressure of 760 mm Hg, is any lung disease present?

Solution: Regarding acidemia, and hypercapnia, the problem should be a respiratory acidosis. Our diagnosis is supported by a normal BE and the bradypnea of the patient. Using Eq. (6.1), we have:

$$\begin{aligned}\Delta\left[\mathrm{HCO_3^-}\right] &= 0.1\,\Delta\, p\mathrm{CO_2} \pm 2 \\ &= 0.1 \times (61-40) \pm 2 \\ &= 2.1 \pm 2\,\mathrm{mEq/L}\end{aligned}$$

Thus, the expected serum $\left[\mathrm{HCO_3^-}\right]$ is from 24.1 to 28.1 mEq/L, which is consistent with the measured value. Therefore, the patient had an acute respiratory acidosis. However, considering the patient's oxygenation, based on what we have learned previously (Chapter 4), the alveolar partial pressure of oxygen can be calculated as:

$$\begin{aligned}p_\mathrm{A}\mathrm{O_2} &= f_\mathrm{i}\mathrm{O_2}\left(p_\mathrm{B} - p_\mathrm{H_2O}\right) - \frac{p_\mathrm{a}\mathrm{CO_2}}{0.8} \\ &= 0.21(760-47) - \frac{61}{0.8} \\ &\approx 150 - 76 \\ &\approx 74\,\mathrm{mm\,Hg}\end{aligned}$$

Thus, the $p_{(\mathrm{A\text{-}a})}\mathrm{O_2}$ is:

$$\begin{aligned}p_{(\mathrm{A\text{-}a})}\mathrm{O_2} &= p_\mathrm{A}\mathrm{O_2} - p_\mathrm{a}\mathrm{O_2} \\ &= 74 - 65 \\ &= 9\,\mathrm{mm\,Hg}\end{aligned}$$

which is within normal limits. Therefore, there is no lung disease present, and the acute respiratory acidosis and hypoxemia are all due to alveolar hypoventilation because of the sedative-induced respiratory center suppression. Providing sufficient ventilation and using the proper antidote will revert all things to normal.

Example Blood gas analysis of a 20-year-old severely ill patient receiving 30% O_2 under a pressure of 760 mm Hg, is reported as follows:

$p\mathrm{CO_2}$ = 40 mm Hg, $\left[\mathrm{HCO_3^-}\right]$ = 23.5 mEq/L, pH = 7.39, BE = −0.74 mEq/L, $p\mathrm{O_2}$ = 95 mm Hg

(a) Does the patient have hypoxemia?
(b) Do we have adequate oxygen transport?
(c) Any evidence suggestive of either hypoventilation or lung disease?

Solution: Regarding the reported values, all measured parameters are normal. With a $p_\mathrm{a}\mathrm{O_2}$ of 95 mm Hg, the patient (breathing 30% O_2) is not hypoxemic. The normal $p\mathrm{CO_2}$ indicates that the alveolar ventilation is normal. However, further information would be needed to assess the adequacy of O_2 transport. If the patient had a normal hemoglobin level and cardiac output, O_2 transport is likely sufficient. Calculating $p_{(\mathrm{A\text{-}a})}\mathrm{O_2}$, we have:

$$\begin{aligned} p_A O_2 &= 0.3(760-47) - \frac{23.5}{0.8} \\ &= 0.3 \times 713 - 29.37 \\ &\approx 185\,\text{mm Hg} \end{aligned}$$

Thus:

$$\begin{aligned} p_{(A\text{-}a)} O_2 &= 185 - 95 \\ &= 90\,\text{mm Hg} \end{aligned}$$

Despite the absence of hypoxemia (p_aO_2 is normal) and alveolar hypoventilation (pCO_2 is normal), the $p_{(A\text{-}a)}O_2$ of 90 mm Hg is abnormally high and clearly reveals an abnormal gas exchange and oxygen transfer in the lung, which in this case is because of severe lung disease. More data are necessary to clarify the nature of the lung disease. It must be noticed that, although the arterial oxygen tension is normal (95 mm Hg), a severe lung disease is diagnosed. This is why the inspired oxygen concentration (f_iO_2) should always be considered.

Example A 47-year-old man with chronic lung disease was brought to the emergency room. On admission, the arterial blood gas values were reported as follows:

pCO_2 = 60 mm Hg, $\left[HCO_3^-\right]$ = 30 mEq/L, pH = 7.320, BE = 3.13 mEq/L, pO_2 = 72 mm Hg (breathing the ambient air with a barometric pressure of 710 mm Hg). What is your diagnosis?

Solution: Considering p_aO_2, and calculating $p_{(A\text{-}a)}O_2$ we have:

$$\begin{aligned} p_A O_2 &= 0.21(710-47) - \frac{60}{0.8} \\ &= 0.21 \times 663 - 75 \\ &\approx 64\,\text{mm Hg} \end{aligned}$$

Thus:

$$\begin{aligned} p_{(A\text{-}a)} O_2 &= 64 - 72 \\ &= -8\,\text{mm Hg} \end{aligned}$$

Having a negative value for $p_{(A\text{-}a)}O_2$, there should be an error in the above information. The patient was either receiving oxygen supplement instead of breathing ambient air, or the reported pCO_2 or p_aO_2 is mistakenly high.

Example A 76-year-old man with gastric outlet obstruction has been undergoing intermittent gastric suction in the last 5 days. The pertinent laboratory values were:

pCO_2 = 49 mm Hg, $\left[HCO_3^-\right]$ = 36 mEq/L, pH = 7.488, BE = 12.33 mEq/L, pO_2 = 67 mm Hg (breathing the ambient air at a barometric pressure of 760 mm Hg), and urinary $[Cl^-]$ = 6 mEq/L. What is the acid-base status?

Solution: Considering the alkalemia, high serum $\left[HCO_3^-\right]$, hypercapnia, and a positive BE, the problem is clearly a metabolic alkalosis. Using Eq. (7.4) (you may prefer to use Eq. (7.5)), then:

$$\begin{aligned}\Delta\, pCO_2 &= (0.4 \text{ to } 0.9)\Delta\left[HCO_3^-\right]\\ &= (0.4 \text{ to } 0.9)\times(36-24)\\ &= (0.4 \text{ to } 0.9)\times 12\\ &= 4.8 \text{ to } 10.8\,\text{mm Hg}\end{aligned}$$

Thus:

$$\begin{aligned}pCO_2 &= 40+(4.8 \text{ to } 10.8)\\ &= 44.8 \text{ to } 50.8\,\text{mm Hg}\end{aligned}$$

Combining what was found and the very low urinary [Cl^-], the diagnosis is a chloride-responsive metabolic alkalosis. Regarding the p_aO_2 and calculating $p_{(A\text{-}a)}O_2$ we have:

$$\begin{aligned}p_AO_2 &= 0.21(760-47)-\frac{49}{0.8}\\ &= 0.21\times 713-61.25\\ &\approx 88\,\text{mm Hg}\end{aligned}$$

Thus:

$$\begin{aligned}p_{(A\text{-}a)}O_2 &= 88-67\\ &= 21\,\text{mm Hg}\end{aligned}$$

This value for $p_{(A\text{-}a)}O_2$ is within the normal range for this age. The patient had a metabolic alkalosis, and in response to this acid-base disturbance he developed a secondary hypoventilation (respiratory compensation for metabolic alkalosis). As a result, the hypoxemia in this patient is entirely due to this secondary hypoventilation, and therefore no lung disease is present.

Example A 54-year-old woman had severe diffuse bilateral pneumonia, ultimately proven to be due to SARS-CoV-2. On admission, she was cyanotic and had a respiratory rate of 50 breaths per minute. Arterial blood gas analysis, while she breathed O_2 via a face mask with an O_2 flow at a rate greater than 15 L/min, revealed:

pCO_2 = 28 mm Hg, $\left[HCO_3^-\right]$ = 20 mEq/L, pH = 7.475, BE = −0.15 mEq/L, pO_2 = 45 mm Hg (barometric pressure of 760 mm Hg)

What is the state of alveolar ventilation and tissue oxygenation in this patient?

Solution: According to alkalemia, hypocapnia, and low serum $\left[HCO_3^-\right]$, the patient had a respiratory alkalosis. The BE is normal, indicating that if the problem was simple, there was an acute process. Employing Eq. (6.3), then:

$$\begin{aligned}\Delta\left[HCO_3^-\right] &= 0.2\,\Delta\, pCO_2 \pm 2\\ &= 0.2\times(40-28)\pm 2\\ &= 2.4\pm 2\,\text{mEq / L}\end{aligned}$$

Therefore, the expected value for serum $\left[HCO_3^-\right]$ ranges from 19.6 to 23.6 mEq/L, which is consistent with the measured plasma $\left[HCO_3^-\right]$. Thus, the patient had an acute respiratory alkalosis. Hypoxemia (p_aO_2 of 45 mm Hg, and cyanosis) was due to severe lung disease. We cannot be sure about the inspired O_2 concentration; we, therefore, cannot calculate the $p_{(A\text{-}a)}O_2$ accurately. Assuming it to be at least 30%, then, we have:

$$\begin{aligned}p_AO_2 &= \frac{30}{100}(760-47)-\frac{28}{0.8}\\ &= 0.3\times 713-35\\ &= 179\,\text{mm Hg}\end{aligned}$$

Thus:

$$\begin{aligned}p_{(A\text{-}a)}O_2 &= 179-45\\ &= 134\,\text{mm Hg}\end{aligned}$$

This abnormally high value indicates a large right-to-left shunt. If the patient does not have any congenital heart diseases, there could be a shunt in the lungs; it might be due to the perfusion of underventilated alveoli, for example. The measured pCO_2 was low, reflecting alveolar hyperventilation in our patient. CO_2 was being washed out from those portions of lung which had an appropriate ventilation and perfusion [5, 6]. This hyperventilation was the cause of the acute respiratory alkalosis.

9.3 Things to Remember

The major causes of hypoxia are $\dot{V}/\dot{Q}$ mismatch, blood shunt, hypoventilation, and diffusion impairment.

Alveolar-arterial pO_2 difference ($p_{(A\text{-}a)}O_2$) is defined as:

$$\begin{aligned}(\text{alveolar-arterial})\ pO_2\ \text{gradient} &= \text{alveolar}\ pO_2 - \text{arterial}\ pO_2\\ p_{(A\text{-}a)}O_2 &= p_AO_2 - p_aO_2\end{aligned}$$

In a normal young person, $p_{(A\text{-}a)}O_2$ averages 8 mm Hg, and linearly increases with age. In hypoxic states which are associated with hypercapnia, a normal $p_{(A\text{-}a)}O_2$ is diagnostic for alveolar hypoventilation; an abnormally high $p_{(A\text{-}a)}O_2$ suggests that a lung disease is also present; a near-zero or negative $p_{(A\text{-}a)}O_2$, in any case, immediately reflects a laboratory error.

There are some important points on the oxyhemoglobin dissociation curve which have clinical values. If $HbO_2\%$ denotes hemoglobin oxygen saturation, these points are:

1. $pO_2 = 20$ mm Hg, $HbO_2\% = 35\%$: a point indicating life-threatening hypoxemia.
2. $pO_2 = 40$ mm Hg, $HbO_2\% = 75\%$: the level at which cyanosis is clearly detectable, provided blood hemoglobin concentration is normal.
3. $pO_2 = 60$ mm Hg, $HbO_2\% = 90\%$: the shoulder of oxyhemoglobin dissociation curve. Below this point the curve is steep.
4. $pO_2 = 80$ mm Hg, $HbO_2\% = 95\%$: normal arterial values for an aged person.
5. $pO_2 = 100$ mm Hg, $HbO_2\% = 97\%$: normal arterial values for a young person.

References

1. West JB. Respiratory physiology. 9th ed. Philadelphia: Lippincott Williams and Wilkins; 2012.
2. Hantzidiamantis PJ, Amaro E. Physiology, alveolar to arterial oxygen gradient. Treasure Island, FL: StatPearls; 2020.
3. Bach J. A quick reference on hypoxemia. Vet Clin North Am Small Anim Pract. 2017;47(2):175–9. https://doi.org/10.1016/j.cvsm.2016.10.004.
4. Ossa Galvis MM, Bhakta RT, Tarmahomed A, Mendez MD. Cyanotic heart disease. Treasure Island, FL: StatPearls; 2020.
5. Singh V, Khatana S, Gupta P. Blood gas analysis for bedside diagnosis. Natl J Maxillofac Surg. 2013;4(2):136–41. https://doi.org/10.4103/0975-5950.127641.
6. Ortiz-Prado E, Dunn JF, Vasconez J, Castillo D, Viscor G. Partial pressure of oxygen in the human body: a general review. Am J Blood Res. 2019;9(1):1–14.

Printed by Printforce, the Netherlands